Living and Coping with Epilepsy, My Way

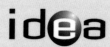

Living and Coping with Epilepsy, My Way

Cara Coles

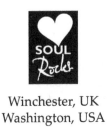

Winchester, UK
Washington, USA

First published by Soul Rocks Books, 2015
Soul Rocks Books is an imprint of John Hunt Publishing Ltd., Laurel House, Station Approach,
Alresford, Hants, SO24 9JH, UK
office1@jhpbooks.net
www.johnhuntpublishing.com
www.soulrocks-books.com

For distributor details and how to order please visit the 'Ordering' section on our website.

Text copyright: Cara Coles 2014

ISBN: 978 1 78279 746 3

A CIP catalogue record for this book is available from the British Library.

Design: Lee Nash

Printed and bound by CPI Group (UK) Ltd, Croydon, CR0 4YY

We operate a distinctive and ethical publishing philosophy in all
areas of our business, from our global network of authors to
production and worldwide distribution.

CONTENTS

This Is Me

Like a lot of people I worked hard and played hard. I worked all the hours I could so that I had money to do all the things I wanted. I thought I was quite happy plodding along with my life, I thought I had my life all mapped out in front of me, but things were about to change.

I was a strong person, someone that could take on anything that life threw at me. I thought I was in control of everything: control to me was good. If I had control of what was going on, nothing could go wrong, but I was soon to find out I was mistaken. There are things in life that are beyond our control.

I was 36 years old, and life was good, a bit of a struggle at times but good, I had control. But it only took a matter of weeks for all this to change and for me to become someone that was:

Fearful – because I didn't know what lay ahead.
Helpless – because I had lost control over my situation and couldn't see any way of regaining it.
Hopeless – because the future looked pretty bleak and I could not see any light on the horizon.

In a matter of a few weeks, my life took a turn I could never have predicted and was turned upside down.

To me routine was everything, I guess getting into a routine makes a busy life easier to juggle; you don't have to think about anything, you just work on auto-pilot. On the morning my life changed for ever, I did the same things I did every morning when I was going to work. I got up, made coffee, put the radio on in the bedroom and put my coffee by the side of the radio. I had turned around to start getting my clothes ready for the day when it happened.

The only way I can describe it is to say that an immense wave of fear swept through my body. The next thing I became conscious of was waking up on the floor: scared, alone, confused, wondering what had just occurred. I got myself back up on my feet and already my mind was working to find a logical reason for what had happened: perhaps I wasn't quite awake, turned too quickly?

I convinced myself that nothing was wrong and carried on with my day as normal. But as the day progressed the pain in my body, every muscle was hurting, became too much. Eventually I had to admit defeat and go home and crawl back into bed.

A few weeks passed and nothing else happened. I decided it must have been a one off event, so I brushed it under the carpet and carried on with life, safe in the belief it wouldn't happen again.

I work in a busy hospital as a registered health care profes-sional and the shifts are often hectic. I had just finished a 12 hour shift and was going on-call. I thought I would just stop and have something to eat before retiring for the night. I remember going into the coffee room and putting my dinner into the microwave. There was another member of staff in the room. We had a brief chat but I had some work to do. I sat down on the chair and turned on the computer. The next thing I knew, I could hear people talking to me, trying to get me to sit back into the chair. I was completely confused and at a loss to understand what had happened. Perhaps, I thought, I had turned too quickly in the chair and, because I had not eaten for a while, I had fainted? From my perspective, that was the only reasonable explanation for finding myself on the floor with no awareness as to how I got there.

Staff were fussing around me, but I couldn't understand why. I had just fainted, that was all. I simply wanted them to leave me alone, there was nothing to worry about and all the fuss was embarrassing. Despite my insistence that I was okay, before I was properly aware of what was going on, I was on a trolley being taken to A&E.

Whilst in A&E some of the department staff where I work called in to see me. "Oh you look better now," they told me. I didn't reply. How could I? I had no idea what had just taken place.

When I saw the doctor he explained that I had experienced a seizure. I tried to explain that I hadn't – I had just fainted. The doctor looked at me and said, "You had a witnessed seizure. Has this happened before?" I explained what had occurred that morning a few weeks ago. The doctor advised me to go and see my GP, which I promised I would. Then I was allowed to go home. I left work feeling somewhat confused. I had suffered a seizure. But how? Why?

It wasn't long before I was sat in front of my GP, who advised me that, because I had now experienced two seizures, my condition was considered problematic and I was not to drive until I had seen the neurologist. He informed me that he would send an urgent request for me to be seen by one.

I went home, went to bed and hid under the duvet. I was scared and confused. I had so many questions; how could I have developed this, what was I going to do? I would lose my driving licence; what about my job? What would I do for a living? But, most importantly, how was I going to cope? There were so many questions running around my head. I don't know how long I cried for but I must have cried myself to sleep.

The next day I went to work and spoke to my boss. Together we decided to remove me off all out of hours work until I had seen the neurologist. I convinced myself this was the first step of losing my job. I had worked so hard to get to where I was today; I left school with no qualifications and joined the royal navy for a brief time. After working in different nursing homes I began working in a busy department. At the age of 29, I finally got a break and was accepted onto a training course. Two years and a lot of hard work later, I became a qualified practitioner. The hard work had continued and two months before the first seizure I had become a senior member of staff.

The job I do is one I had dreamt about for years but had never thought it would be possible. When I left school with nothing, I honestly thought that my working life would consist of menial jobs without any prospect of changing that. However, with hard work I had proved myself wrong and now I feared I was going to lose it all.

Before I had even begun to come to terms with things, I found myself sat in front of the neurologist. There is a lot of what he said to me that I don't remember. I do remember him explaining that it sounded like I was having tonic-clonic seizures. He wanted me to have tests before he started me on any medications, and I would have to surrender my driving licence to the DVLA. He could have said anything after that, but all I could focus on was that I wouldn't be able to drive any more.

I went home in shock. I had just been diagnosed with epilepsy without being given any information about what to expect or how to deal with it. For the first time in my life I felt completely alone. I had tons of questions and no one to ask them of.

I wrote the hardest letter I had ever had to write in my life, a letter to the DVLA, explaining why I was sending my driving licence to them. I'm surprised there weren't tear stains on the paper. As I wrote I felt that my life, all that I knew, everything I was, was falling apart. I posted the letter with no idea when, or if, I would ever see my driving licence again.

My head was constantly full of questions; what was causing this, how long would it go on for? Even more importantly, when would it happen next? The questions kept coming but not the answers. So I turned to the internet and most of the information I have gained is from there. I discovered a great website called, 'Epilepsy Action', as well as some other excellent sites. As I began researching, I was shocked by how little I understood about epilepsy, and in time I started to find out how little knowledge other people had. I began to realize there was a need to make people more aware of the condition. My own experiences had left me scared and confused, and although I had wonderful friends and family, I felt so alone without anyone to answer my questions.

I have made many mistakes in my life, but not talking to people about how I felt and how I was coping, or rather, not coping, during this time was one big mistake. I felt that if I could hide my real feelings about it all from my family and friends, they wouldn't see how much I was hurting, how scared I was, how much I had lost control of my life.

Then the tests started. I remember lying in the MRI scanner, trying to keep still. "Don't cry," I told myself. "Don't cry." I could feel the tears rolling down my cheeks. What if there was something in my brain causing this? What if there was nothing? Surely someone of 36 doesn't just develop epilepsy? What if there was something wrong with my brain? The scan was clear and so were all the other tests.

It was such a relief. Still in a state of shock over it all, I thought that was it. My scan was clear, no more seizures. By the time I saw the neurologist again I had already had another seizure and so I started medication.

I tried to deal with life as best as I could, but I think I was just going through the motions. Just plodding along, trying to keep going, pretending everything was okay. I put on a mask, a brave face, so that nobody could see what was going on inside me.

The next major hurdle I had to face was what to do with my car. It had been sat in the car park for a while now. With no driving licence, there was only one thing I could do and that was to sell it. As I handed the keys and documents over to the new owner, and watched them drive away, I watched my freedom drive away with them. I never thought that this would happen to me. I can't even start to explain how much it hurt.

I bought myself a Medic-alert bracelet. I appreciated they

saved people lives but I hated wearing it. It felt as if I was being labelled. Looking back, I think it was because I still didn't believe it. My friends and family were brilliant, and work was amazing, but I still felt like my life was falling apart.

I decided to put a face on, show the world I could deal with this. But it was all a front, deep down I couldn't get past the idea that my life was falling apart. Even though I had all these people giving me support, I felt so alone, no one to talk to that understood. How was I going to deal with this? What caused it? Was it ever going to stop? Not knowing what was going to happen was hard for me to deal with.

I found myself giving up so much, all because I had epilepsy: my driving licence, my independence. I gave up so many things that I enjoyed doing. It seemed as if everything I looked at, all I could see was, 'I cannot do that, what if I have a seizure'. The fear of having a seizure was taking over my whole life.

So this is me. I have epilepsy, and, back then, at that moment in time, my life was crashing down around me and I was powerless to stop it.

What Changed

I have an interest in the paranormal, mainly in the subject of ghosts. I enjoy the research side of things, and trying to understand why some people see and hear things that most of us are completely unaware of, and that some would deny exist. This was one of the many things I had given up due to the epilepsy, but I needed to get my teeth into something, to take my mind of what was happening.

One day I found myself reading a piece in a magazine about the law of attraction. The thought that I could have anything I wanted was tantalizing, now more than ever. This, I thought, is what I need to get my teeth into. I couldn't wait to know more, I wanted to know if it was really possible. As I delved into it further, I began to understand that everything is made of energy, even our thoughts have energy. What we think, we can create. What we feel, we attract and what we imagine, we will become.

From that first article I bought a book, and then another. Before long I had quite a collection. I turned the idea that I could really have anything I wanted over and over in my mind. One part of me just didn't believe it; surely, it couldn't be true? How could someone like me have whatever they wanted? The more I read though, the more confused I got. One book would tell me one thing, and then another would tell me to do it differently. Other books were telling me what I was doing was wrong and that I should be using a different method.

I have no idea how much I spent on books on this subject, yet still in the back of my mind I couldn't believe that I could have all I wanted. I was reading the books and the examples of people getting what they wanted and these things seemed to just happen. But surely they had to do something towards fulfilling their wish; things don't just fall into place so you can get everything you want. Surely we have to work towards things, that's what I was always told. You worked hard to get what you want.

Most of the examples showed what people wished for and the end result, but not the in between bits. To me the in between bits are important. A bald statement of what people wanted and wished for and an equally bald statement that they got their wish wasn't enough for me. I needed to know if they did anything to help them achieve their wish or if they simply put the wish out there, sat back and it appeared. So many questions, and I had so little proof that it worked, yet all these people were saying it did. I just needed to see one person's account of *how* it worked for them, to truly believe.

I had been so busy researching the law of attraction that, at some point, I had stopped questioning why I got epilepsy, and in fact, I had stopped focusing on what I had lost. So there was only one thing for me to do and that was to put the law of attraction to the test.

This book is my journey, living with epilepsy, the highs as well as the lows. How I used the law of attraction to help me overcome and deal with my illness. In this book I share the situations I went through and what I discovered to help me deal with it all in the best way. You may have just been diagnosed or you may have had epilepsy for a while. You may be reading this because a loved one has been diagnosed. You may even have been diagnosed with another illness. I hope, whatever the circumstances are that bring you here, that you all find this book to be helpful.

Accepting Your Illness

It wasn't until later on in the project that I learnt to accept that I had epilepsy. Perhaps it was something I should have addressed earlier than I did. You have to accept that you have this, or any other illness. Although you can't accept it overnight, you will have to accept that you will have to make changes to your life and this can be hard. You may need to allow yourself time to grieve for your past life. I grieved for my driving licence, my loss of independence; I grieved because I was diagnosed with epilepsy.

There are so many different types of epilepsy that I can't do the whole subject justice here. If you want to learn more, please look at the Epilepsy Action website. It's full of wonderful information.

There are so many things that have to be taken into account that people often don't realize, like possibly working out financial issues, managing medication, transport issues. Someone who suffers from epilepsy has to learn to look at things differently and to think about their safety. At the end of a working day, I used to love having a bath; it was a great way to relax. Once the seizures started, I felt it was unsafe to have a bath when I was alone in the house; there was always the risk that I could have a seizure in the bath. So instead, I would make my husband stand outside the bathroom door and keep talking: not very relaxing, so showers from then on.

Look at sharp edges on furniture, something I didn't think about until I had a seizure and hit my head against a bedside cabinet. I think I failed to consider my safety because I hadn't yet accepted that I had epilepsy. You know better than anyone about your seizures, so please just have a look around your home and see if there are changes you need to make to keep you safe. You can do whatever you want to do with your life, but you need to make sure you are safe should you have a seizure.

There may be occasions when you experience loneliness, embarrassment and even fear. It takes time to adjust and it takes longer to accept. But eventually, if you want to achieve your dreams, you do need to accept your illness. You have to come to terms with your limitations and learn how to accommodate them, developing new skills and ways to help you to cope with your illness.

Grief when you are diagnosed is normal; don't think you are alone, talk to people, whether a professional or your family and friends. Be open with your family and friends, and remember, they may need time to adjust to your diagnosis and it may help if you talk about it together. But please, talk to someone, I made the mistake of thinking I could deal with everything alone, a decision that I would later regret.

When I was first told I had epilepsy I felt like everything was slipping away, any control I'd had, had been taken away from me. I felt as if I had lost the person I once was, lost my real self. It is important to remember that epilepsy is part of you, it's not who you are. Learn about your illness, is there anything you can do to minimize its impact; change your diet, increase your exercise levels. Look at ways to help you gain control over your life. Just because you have an illness it does not mean that you have to let it control you. Too many times I have seen people just accepting their illness and not being willing to do anything for themselves. They almost become their illness and let it control their whole lives.

I'm hoping, as you read the rest of this book, that you will gain strength from it and that the information and ideas it contains will help you as they helped me. You don't have to believe in the law of attraction but there are things that I'm passing on to you that really helped me deal with living with epilepsy and I hope they will help others to gain what they want out of life.

If you take anything away from this book, let it be the fact that:

you have an illness: that doesn't mean you *are* that illness. It's still your life: how you live it is up to you. You are who you are; you are not what your illness says you are.

The Project

The law of attraction, can we truly believe that there is a force that can help us to gain what we want out of life, or is it just a great story? For me there was only one thing to do – put the law of attraction to the test. Problem was, I had no clue how I was going to do that.

Then I had an idea. I would live my life according to the law of attraction for a year, from January 2010 to January 2011. It couldn't be that difficult, right? Actually, there was a lot more to it than I thought, but once I had got to grips with the basics it wasn't that difficult to do. What took me longest was trying to get my head around all the different ideas I had read from different books. It would have been a whole lot easier if I had just stuck to one book. But hey, why make life simpler? Eager to start the project, I bought myself a notebook. My plan was to write down everything that happened during that year, all my achievements, ideas and things I had learnt along the way.

Making notes along the journey was a great idea and I'm so glad I did. It's a good idea for everyone, but even more so if you have epilepsy because some of us forget things along the way. Reading back on the notes I made prior to writing this book has been interesting. I had forgotten some of the things that had happened during that year and it was a pleasant surprise to rediscover them when reading back. It was also interesting to see how much I had changed during that time, and, as I read the notes, I saw I had been slowly heading towards my goals.

Your notes are personal, nobody has to read them, so you are free to write whatever you want, don't hold back. When you read your notes remember, it's not just about seeing the big changes in your life, notice the small things as well. Sometimes it's the small things that mean the most and perhaps lead you to your desired dream. So every now and then have a look through your note book and see the changes that have taken place. In retrospect you may notice small changes in your life that at the time you missed.

Writing notes really helped whilst I was having seizures. They helped to give me a focus, a reason to keep going. I knew I had a future to look forward to because seeing what I had already achieved gave me a major boost and made me want to carry on. Of course I needed to decide what it was I wanted out of life, something I had not thought about for some time. This turned out to be quite hard, harder than I had initially imagined. I sat there for a quite a while, trying to work out what it was I really wanted, no point carrying on with the project if I couldn't decide that.

So get your notebooks out and start to think about what it is you want. If you could have anything in the world, what would that be? Once you have decided, write it down. Write whatever comes to mind, even if it sounds silly or impossible.

My Wishes

Now for the fun part, because now you get to decide what it is you really want for your future. You may already know what it is you want or, like me, have no idea at all. I soon saw that before my seizures I was just plodding along. I had worked hard for the career that I have, but since then I had just been stuck in a rut with no direction. There was a period from when my seizures started until I began this project, almost a year in fact, where I allowed the epilepsy to take over. Let's call that my grief period, my time of trying to cope with all the sudden changes that the illness brought with it. That year was pretty tough, in more ways than one. It was towards the end of the year that I started to read about the law of attraction. The more I read, the more I wanted to know. I was ready to get my life back. It was time to stop plodding along and to start living.

However, the big question still remained. What did I want out of life; what did I want out of this project apart from helping others? A couple of months before I decided to start the project we lost one of our beloved dogs. We still had a dog, and I thought it was time to look to get another, at the time it was only a thought. As we re-home dogs the thought of going around rescue centres didn't fill me with much joy, if I could, I would have taken them all home. So when I started to write my wishes for this project that was the first thing I put on there. Another dog that would get along with the little lady we already had. What was the chance that a few days later I would get a phone call asking if we would consider taking in another dog? Of course we did, and he is a wonderful addition to our family. It was amazing and I was somewhat blown away by it. Was there really a possibility that we can all have whatever we want?

After this event I took a hard look at my life and tried to decide what it was I really wanted. It was while I was thinking about what I truly wanted that I thought about writing this book. I had no idea what was going to happen, but there was this urge to write this book. So I went with my gut feeling and, with pen in hand, started to write notes in my notebook about what was happening. I had no idea where it was going to take me, but I had an urge to share my story in the hope that it would help others. I wanted to show people that there is light at the end of the tunnel and to prove that you can have what you want out of life, epilepsy doesn't have to stop you from experiencing life to the fullest. It's all there if you want it.

With note book in hand, I stared at the blank page for a while. I seemed to sit there for a long time, and still no idea what I really wanted. I could have asked for more money, my dream house. But isn't that what we all want? No, it had to be something different, something that would blow my mind and leave me in no doubt that the law of attraction does in fact work. In the end I imagined a genie standing in front of me, granting me five wishes.

This is what I came up with:

My first wish was to be seizure free and to have my driving licence by the time the project was completed.

The second was that, although I love my job in health care and will continue to progress further in my career; I also wanted to start working from home more. When I wrote that wish that was what I wanted. Things have since changed.

My third wish, having never won a competition, was to win some of the competitions I entered so that I could share the prizes I won with family and friends.

Before I had even started the project things changed. My first wish, well that wasn't going to be, I had one seizure in the

January and then another in the March. But I wasn't giving up. I wasn't going to let that put me off the project. I decided instead to change the project start date to April and I changed the date of my wish, to have my driving licence back, to the end of the project in April 2011.

It was my chance, and now it's your chance, to dream big. Get that notebook out and write down everything that you want out of life, don't hold back, just let your pen flow. Write whatever feels right for you, it doesn't matter what others think. What matters is what *you* want. What is it that you enjoy; where do you want to go with your life. Take a chance; you have nothing at all to lose and everything to gain.

I still had two more wishes. Wish number four was all about this book. I wanted to be published. Not self-published, but published by a company. That way the achievement of my wish was taken out of my hands. After all, it wouldn't have been much of a test to wish for the book to be published to prove that the law of attraction works and then simply to publish the book myself. I was quite specific when phrasing this particular wish. I wrote down, 'in order to prove that the law of attraction works, this book is going to be published by a publishing company'.

Then I thought, well surely I should have a few more wishes, this doesn't seem like much. I wanted something else, something bigger, something that was going to blow my mind. Perhaps something that I could not achieve no matter how hard I might work at making it happen. After hours of thinking, my eyes lit upon one particular object in the house and in that split second I knew what my main wish was going to be.

Dream Big

This is your chance to really dream big; don't be afraid to do so. It is your life; so what you wished for sounds crazy to everyone else, so what? If it is going to make you happy, just go for it. At the end of the day you are responsible for making your own happiness. You are not here just to make other people happy. Selfish? Perhaps, but while you have to take into account other people in your life, you can't live only to make them content.

It doesn't matter what you do, people will always be ready to comment on your choices. That's okay. Freedom of speech is a good thing. Freedom of choice is even better. Let them comment – just remember to ignore them. People lined up to tell me I was crazy when they heard what I had planned; in fact, they had a lot more than that to say. Most of what they had to say was about my last, most important, wish.

At the end of the day, we all have to go on our own little adventures to find out who we really are and where we belong. This is my adventure, the first of many. It is my way of re-discovering myself. My life has changed thanks to the epilepsy and now I'm taking control and changing my life again, on my terms this time. So when you read my last wish I hope you will understand why I went for it.

After each seizure I would have memory problems. That split second when you wake up on the floor, no idea where you are, you may be in your own home, but for that split second, you could be anywhere. Then once you have calmed down you may realize you are in your bedroom. On one occasion an ambulance was called, and the ambulance crew kept talking to me, asking me questions that I couldn't answer. I could only just about remember my name let alone what medication I'm on or what day it was.

I was half way to the hospital before I realized I'd had a

seizure. In time, slowly, my memory starts to come back. But it takes a little while before I can remember the names of simple, everyday objects. For quite a few hours it's like playing charades. I try to act out what it is I want, whilst moving about as little as possible because any form of movement hurts like anything. I can see what I want in my mind, but can't remember what the item is called. Normally, after a good sleep, my memory comes back fully.

You also become expert at dealing with everyday memory problems. Smart phones are great because you set alarms for when to take your tablets and for any appointments you may have. I carry a note book around so I can write notes as I'm going through the day; I have been known to set an alarm to remind myself to check the note book! It's one of the side effects that a lot of us with epilepsy have to work out ways to deal with.

Over time I saw my memory problem was in fact worse than I thought. I had come to terms with the day to day memory problems, only to realize I was finding it hard to remember things from my past. I would be talking to someone and they would say, "Do you remember when?" I would give them a confused look because I didn't remember the event. At first I ignored it, putting it down to one of those things. Then a little while later I would be talking to someone else, "Do you remember going to?" At first I tried to hide the fact I couldn't remember some of the things people would talk about, but when it kept happening, I had to admit it, there were things in my life I didn't remember.

It's a bit like something has just come along and erased snippets of my past. Worst of all, almost after every seizure, a little bit more of my past has been erased. After a while people stopped saying, "Do you". Instead they would say, "Surely you remember when", as if whatever they were talking about was some major event in my life. But I didn't have any recollection of it. They would show me pictures, but not even those could jog my memory. Whatever it was had been completely erased from my memory.

What did I do? Well, now I was trying to hide the fact that, not only was I scared of the seizures and the pain, now I was also scared of how much of my past memory I would end up losing. At this point, it's important to mention that not everyone with epilepsy has the same memory difficulties. Not every person with epilepsy will have the same side effects. Also, some memory problems can be a side effect of the anti-epileptic drugs, rather than of the illness itself. If you are worried talk to your doctor about any problems you may be experiencing.

In the summer of 2009, I was out with my best friend; we were having a laugh about our favourite band. They were going back to the studio to write an album. A new album would mean a tour. While we were out shopping we saw some saving tins and decided that from that moment we would collect every two pound coin we got, to put into our saving tins, so that when the boys toured we would be able to go to all of their concerts. Neither of us had done this before, so why not. I came home the proud owner of a saving tin. Excitedly, I placed it in a prime location. We had no idea when the album was coming, or even if they were going to tour.

Whilst racking my brain for my ultimate, amazing wish for the project, I found myself sitting there, looking at the saving tin one day. That led me to thinking about my past. I was reminiscing about some of the concerts I had been to. In particular I was trying to remember my first ever concert, to see the band we were saving up to go and see on tour. I couldn't, I could recollect waiting for the coach with my school friend and that was it. I could remember where the concert was, but I couldn't call to mind arriving at the venue, there was nothing about the concert itself, or what happened after it finished.

In a slight state of panic I thought about other things I could summon up concerning the band. I could think back to the very first album of theirs I had been given, along with my first record player. Oh yes, I did remember that so well. I could even recollect the overwhelming emotions I had when I opened the present. I also recalled that we were at my grandparents that Christmas, and I had to wait until we got home before I could play the album. As a teenager that was punishment by parents, I could remember how my room looked in the 80s with posters all over the place. But I couldn't bring to mind that concert. Going to their first concert is a big event in someone's life, but for me it had been completely erased. As I sat staring at the saving tin, a thought popped into my head; stop stressing out about what you can't remember and look to make a new memory. A new memory of something I never thought it would be possible to achieve. So with that thought in mind, I got my notebook out and wrote my last wish for my project.

My best friend and I are going to meet the band. Oh yes – you read that right.

I wrote it down; put it out to the universe, simply saying, "Here you go! Now blow my mind! I leave the when and where up to you"

That may sound crazy to some, but it was perfect. With my last, ultimate, amazing wish decided on, I soon stopped thinking about all the events I had forgotten about. Now I had a new focus. It was just what I needed to deal with my memory problem. I had managed to stop stressing out about it: turned it around and was ready to set about making new memories. This was the big wish that would blow my mind. It was also a total long shot. Such a long shot that, if it happened, there would be no doubt in my mind that the law of attraction really did work.

So I had my wishes, my excitement was high. Now it was time for me to stop wishing my life away and to make those wishes happen.

What We Attract Into Our Lives

The first thing I started to get my head around was, *like attracts like*. This is something that will keep coming up. Everything is made of energy, and we attract the same energy that we give out. Our thoughts are energy, our actions are energy and our feelings are energy. The energy that we send out is what will return into our lives.

So if we think and feel more positive, we will attract more positive things into our lives. On the other hand if we think and feel negative about ourselves then we will attract negative things into our lives. So being happy attracts more happiness and happy things happen to us, but the reverse is also true. Being sad attracts more sadness into your life. Sounds simple, doesn't it? But I'm going to be honest. I had problems getting my head around it, because when I first started to look at, *like attracts like*, I started to think, if we attract everything into our lives, does that mean I attracted epilepsy? The question went over and over in my head. I looked to books and websites for help with an answer. Some would say, 'It's a test' or 'It's not so much that you attract these things but it's how you deal with them that's important'. "Okay," I told myself, "I can deal with that." The trouble was, instead of accepting those answers I carried on looking. I came across a website saying things like, 'If you get sick or hurt, it's all your own fault. You attract these things into your life'. I didn't read the rest. In fact I stopped looking altogether.

Personally, I could not believe that people attract illness into their lives. But having seen that website, the idea went over and over in my mind. The whole notion started to get me down; in the end I had to give myself a talking to. "No," I told myself. "I did not attract this." I most certainly don't want anyone else to get the impression that they attracted an illness into their lives. The best thing to do is to accept it's happened and focus on finding a way to deal with it. For myself, I knew I had to draw a line under the situation and move on with my life, and that's what I did. It is not easy accepting this condition, but I have to, we all have to, we need to move on. Worrying about how or why this happened or what, if anything, we did to bring this into our lives causes nothing but more worry and stress and, no-one, ill or well, needs any more of that in their daily living. I stopped looking at how or if I had attracted epilepsy, and I stopped looking for a reason why it started at the age of 36. It was time to accept I had epilepsy, and that I had it for life. I had to keep thinking, one day these seizures will stop. We need to keep reminding ourselves that epilepsy is a part of us, it doesn't control us. Accepting that you have epilepsy doesn't happen overnight, it will take time. Take each day as it comes.

So now you have drawn a line under whatever it is you have. You've looked at using *like attracts like*, and how that can help you to achieve what you want out of life. It's time now to change your thoughts and change your life. There are those who say we need to become what it is we want to attract. Your thoughts, your actions, your emotions are all energy – vibrations that you are sending out. What I send out I shall receive. This sounds very much like Karma, a subject I'm sure we have all heard about. You get what you give. Causing suffering to others will cause suffering to you. Causing happiness to others will result in happiness for you.

Simply put, you attract into your life whatever you give your energy, focus and attention to, whether wanted or unwanted, consciously or unconsciously. This means you can have anything you want, no matter how big or how crazy it may seem.

- You reap what you sow.
- What goes around comes around.
- Good creates good.

If I say kind words to you, this may result in your feeling peaceful and happy. If I say harsh words to you, you could be upset and hurt. This kindness or harshness will return to me, through others, at a later time. When I looked at the world like this, I soon recognized how I was treating others. Soon afterwards I started to notice how other people were treating others. I was shocked, but I could not say anything; it was not my place to.

Raising your vibrations will make you feel good about yourself. You are the author of your life, no-one else. How you live, how you act, and react to others is all up to you. You can change your life; the only thing stopping you is yourself. You need to want to change and to believe that you can.

Like attracts like, happiness attracts happiness, love attracts love, respect attracts respect. On the other hand, sadness attracts sadness. Everything you do in your life attracts the same back, this applies to actions, feelings, and even your own thoughts. You will find that like attracts like will keep coming up in other areas, so this is an important subject to think about.

A few things to keep in mind.

- Learn to love yourself a little bit more each day.
- Be kind and look for the best in everyone.
- Show respect to everyone you encounter.
- Don't be cruel with your words.
- Smile more and frown less.
- Expect life to be good and you'll have everything you need and want from life.
- Always believe something wonderful is about to happen.

It doesn't happen overnight, and it may seem hard to believe but changing how you think can really change your life. Every single thing you do is sending a message out to the universe, so make sure that what you are sending out is what you want to receive.

Some things you just have to face. It is very difficult, but there are times when you have to face your fears. Why do we fear things? Often it is because something occurred in childhood or in your teenage years or adult life that was traumatic and left you fearful of the same or similar situations arising again. Some people believe that you bring your issues with you from a past life. Whatever you believe in, all of us have some kind of anxiety.

Fear can help to protect you as it alerts you to possible danger. The fight or flight response is the body preparing itself to deal with perceived danger. There are so many fears, too many to mention them all here.

If you want to progress to achieving what you want then you have to face your issues. Although, as already mentioned, fears and anxieties are common in everyone's lives; it's how we deal with them that is important. For those of us who have epilepsy, our qualms can focus on having a seizure, or having a seizure in front of strangers. That concern alone is sometimes enough to stop us from doing things we secretly long to do. Some of us avoid going to public places or using public transport because of the worry of having a seizure. In extreme cases people become afraid of leaving the safety of their home.

Any loss of independence is hard to take and I did struggle to accept that my life had changed. Living with unpredictable seizures is very difficult. Having to accept that you may have to make changes to your life to stay safe is hard. It can help to talk to people, family, friends, or professionals, they may have ideas on how to strike a balance between keeping safe and allowing ourselves some independence. You may have epilepsy but you don't have to go through everything alone. Accepting help makes you no lesser a person. Remember, it's important to recognize that epilepsy is a part of your life but it doesn't control your life.

People tend to avoid the situation or things they are scared of. This doesn't help them overcome their agitation, in fact, it can be the reverse. Avoiding something scary reinforces your anxiety, making it stronger. My concern is: what if we are missing out on things because our apprehensiveness stops us from leaving our comfort zone? Could we be missing opportunities to achieving our dreams? How can we show the universe that we really want these dreams to be fulfilled if we are busy hiding behind our worries and not prepared to step out of our comfort zones?

People can overcome their alarm by exploring and gradually getting used to the thing or the situation they are afraid of. I have some friends who dread flying and I admire them because, although they find it difficult, they still fly. Their mind set is that if they want to go abroad they cannot let their consternation get in the way. Remember, you don't have to face your fears alone, ask friends or family for help, or even seek professional help. It's your choice, you don't have to face anything you don't want to; nobody can make you do something you don't want to do. All I can say is that facing a fear can be such an uplifting experience.

Living in a small village can make getting around difficult. Thankfully there is a train station. To keep as much independence as I could I would have to catch the train. My family and friend were amazing and offered to drive me places, which was great. I'm not sure that they understood, but I needed to do as much as I could for myself. I could catch the train to work, or to visit the doctor, and to do a bit of shopping. At first I hated it. I was scared, what if I had a seizure on the train or on the platform. Armed with my medic-alert on my wrist, I would go off. Then, one day, I thought my worst nightmare was about to happen.

I was sat at the busy train station waiting to go home when an intense fear washed over me. I started to find it difficult to breathe. I was hot and dizzy and very scared. My legs were becoming weak. I managed to find a seat and started to try and slow my breathing down. I kept saying to myself over and over again, "Please not here." It felt like a life time, but it wasn't long before the feeling started to go. I was so glad to make it home and put the experience behind me. Then a week later it happened again. I sat there terrified that I was going to have a seizure on the platform but I calmly talked myself out of it and the feeling passed.

I spoke to my neurologist about these odd attacks I was having. He listened and then asked me when they happened. Then he told me that the attacks were nothing to do with my epilepsy. They were in fact panic attacks. I was kind of relieved, but then I thought, how do I overcome this?

Panic attacks are periods of intense fear that are of sudden onset. I very much hope that this doesn't happen to you but here is what to look out for if it does. This is a list of some of the main symptoms.

- A sensation that your heart is beating irregularly.
- Hot or cold flushes and sweating.
- Trembling.
- Shortness of breath.
- Chest pain.
- Feeling sick.
- You may feel an overwhelming sense of fear and a sense of unreality, as if you're detached from the world around you.

If you are breathing quickly during a panic attack, slowing your breathing down can ease your other symptoms.

- Cup your hands together over your mouth and nose or use a paper bag – but never a plastic bag.
- Breathe deeply through your nose.
- Breathe out slowly through your mouth.
- Focus your thinking on the word 'calm'.

Keep calm and concentrate on your breathing. You should start to feel better as the level of carbon dioxide in your blood returns to normal.

If you are with someone who is having a panic attack, reassure them that it will soon pass and the symptoms are nothing to worry about. Keep them calm and if need be, clear the area around them.

So now I was having panic attacks simply because I was scared of having a seizure in front of people, I'm guessing you can't get much busier than a train station at peak times. At this point I could not decide what to do. There was the fear of catching the train and the tiredness from the medication, yet I could not sleep at night because I dreaded waking up on the floor. All of this was starting to get to me. I realized I had to face all of it if I wanted to get my life back together.

Now when I left the house I was armed with my medic-alert bracelet and a paper bag. I took the train to work or to do some shopping whenever I could. As time went by, the panic attacks stopped.

I started to look at my other qualms. I have always been apprehensive about talking in public. I invariably sat at the back in lectures or shows, in case I was asked questions or asked for my opinion. But as my wishes for my future started to change, I knew I might have to do more public speaking. I don't know how the anxiety started and it may never leave me, but I will face up to it when the time comes. Nothing is going to stop me from gaining what I want for my future.

Many years ago, I had a fear of joining new groups and meeting new people. The thought of entering a room full of strangers, all looking at you as you walked through the door, would really put me off doing things. I went through a period in my life where I felt I wasn't good enough and was worried that I was going to be judged. On the other hand, I had a real interest in paranormal research. At the time it was an area I understood little about and there is only so much you can learn from books, I understood if I wanted to find out more about research I would have to join a group. There are times when nothing is better than learning from other people.

So I joined groups like the 'Ghost Club' and 'ASSAP'. From there I joined a local group, where I met my best friend. Then we started our own group. So I soon got over my initial worries, but the dread of talking in public remained and I would always let someone else take up that role. Of course that has now changed, I know now that I can face the fear of talking in public. Not only that, but if I was going to achieve my wish to meet the band, I would have to get over my apprehension in order to talk to them.

Instead of giving in to your anxieties and letting them control you, you can use them in a more positive way, you can use them to drive you. Facing what you fear can not only help you to achieve the things you want, it is also guaranteed to give you a great feeling when you have overcome whatever you were fearful of. You did it! You started to overcome something that was holding you back in some way, and that is such a positive thing. If you can face your distress, surely, you can face anything?

There is a wealth of information out there about overcoming fear. It is of course up to you if you want to take up this help but, assuming you do, you would be wise to invest some time in researching the different methods to see what might work best for you. It isn't a given that what worked for one will definitely work for another and you might have to try out a few different approaches before you find the right one for you.

Don't let a few fears keep you from making your dreams come true.

Let Your Imagination Run Wild

Visualization is a technique that uses your imagination to help make your dreams into reality. Used in the right way, creative visualization can improve your life and attract success and prosperity. It can help you to achieve your goals. Goals and aspirations give us a direction in life. Mine have given me hope for the future.

By visualizing a certain event, situation or object, such as a car, a house, or meeting a band, in vivid detail, carefully including every tiny aspect, you attract it into your life. Visualization is a process that is similar to daydreaming. There are people who use this technique naturally in their everyday lives, consciously or unconsciously, attracting the success they want by visualizing their goals as already accomplished. So for myself, I visualise people reading this book, I visualise talking to the band, I also visualise my future in a positive way. As I'm writing this, my favourite song by the band has started playing on the radio. Little things like this help me not only to visualize the event but also to inject greater feeling into my desire to make my wish real. It's important that you add as much as you can to your visualization. It's not just about seeing things happen in your mind; you also need to try to add some emotion.

Have fun with your visualization; see it as a movie and you are the star of the show. Have music playing, add colour, feel the emotion of achieving your goal. Make your visualization feel real, because soon it will be. For example, if you want more money, imagine how you would feel if you had it. What you would do with it? How happy would you be? Allow yourself 10 to 30 minutes every day, or at least every other day, for visualizing your goals. Set aside time to rest and remove yourself from everything else going on. Find a quiet, uninterrupted area to practice the technique. Remember, the more you focus on your goals, the sooner you will achieve them. I know finding time is not always easy, if I don't get time during the day, I quite often visualise my goals as I go off to sleep, that way I know I won't be interrupted.

I have also been known to do my visualizing on the train station while waiting for the train home. Although it's not quiet, by focusing on my wishes it takes my mind off what is going on around me. It's an excellent way to stop me thinking about my fear of having a seizure. One thing to remember though is to keep an eye on the time. Once or twice I was so busy day dreaming that I nearly missed my train.

Only visualize positive events and ones that are not going to hurt you or anyone else. Remember, like attracts like. There may be times when you find that while you are doing your visualization some negative thoughts creep in. When this happens to me, I stop what I'm doing and do something else to take my mind of the negative thoughts. Then I make a point of doing some visualization later on in the day when I'm thinking more positively. It is important to maintain positivity when visualizing.

Here are a few things which may help you with your visualization techniques.

Vision Boards

Vision boards are a great tool to aid in manifesting your goals and dreams. They help you to keep focused. How you arrange your boards is up to you, use pictures, words and colour. Anything that makes you feel good and that is connected to your wishes.

The board is there as a reminder to you of what you want in your life. It's a great way to make you feel good and images are a great way to help you with your visualization. Let yourself be excited as you arrange your board because you are creating your future.

There is plenty of different advice out there on what to make your board out of, or where you should place it. Some sources advise putting a finished board away where you cannot see it. The idea is that this sends a message to the universe that you trust your dream is being dealt with and you are also not monitoring its progress. Other sources advise the complete opposite, saying that keeping your vision board where it is visible is a great daily reminder of what it is you want out of life.

As I see it, a vision board is a very personal thing, so you will have to choose what to do. If you do want to use it as a daily reminder then place it somewhere out of general public view. Have a go at making one and see what feels good for you. By all means read all the advice on what to make it out of, but ultimately, what you decide to do with your board is up to you. The board is an aid to help you. For me it worked, it helped me to focus my mind when things got on top of me. However, you may decide you don't need one. That's fine. It's whatever works for you that is important.

My vision board is made out of cork. I chose cork because I can easily pin things to it and change things around, as well as adding things when I feel like it. I don't see that there is any harm in updating it, as it keeps the energy connection strong and fresh. I look out for examples and information which I can then add to the board, or, when a wish is fulfilled, I can easily change my board to reflect a different goal. It can be fun looking and searching for images for it. Even after all this time I still find myself searching through magazines for possible pictures or articles. I keep my board by the side of my bed, so that I can see it when I wake up and last thing before I go to sleep. It helps me with my practice last thing at night.

My vision board has helped me to sustain focus even when I'm exhausted. If you have epilepsy you will know what I mean when I talk about the tiredness you feel after a seizure. It's hard to describe, but you just want to sleep. It feels as if someone has come along and sapped all your energy. There is also the post-seizure pain to deal with. It feels as if every muscle in my body hurts, any movement makes me cry out as the pain is so bad. Often the best way for me to manage this is to try to get to sleep before the pain starts.

In the May of 2010, I had a seizure. I woke up on the floor by the side of my bed. At the time I didn't know what had happened and couldn't understand why my husband had called an ambulance. The paramedic was talking to me, but all I could really do was look at him. I could hear what he was saying but it didn't make sense. It didn't help that he was asking me lots of questions which I could not answer. The confusion after this seizure seemed to take quite a while to clear. I was halfway to the hospital before I started to realize I was in an ambulance, then it began to dawn on me that I had had a seizure, although I still couldn't understand why my husband had called an ambulance. The problem is that when you have a seizure, you have no idea of what is happening, which, as far as I'm concerned is a good thing. However, I had no idea that as I fell out of bed, I had hit the bedside cabinet. I had taken a chunk out of the side of my nose and I had a large cut on my right eyebrow and later I developed a beautiful black eye.

After spending hours in A&E being patched up, I didn't get to bed till after the post-seizure pain had started, which was making it impossible to get to sleep. I was feeling very low. I lay in bed and just looked at my vision board. I couldn't remember what anything was called that was pinned on there but it didn't seem to matter. I felt calm looking at all the things I'd put onto it. It gave me a sense that everything was going to be okay. Having the board there helped me to focus on what I wanted for the future and not on the pain and the fact that I had experienced another seizure. Soon I dropped off to sleep.

The vision boards not only help with visualization, they can also help you to focus on what you want for your future, even in difficult times.

Vision Books

As well as a vision board, I also have a vision book. I like to call it my dream book. In my book I have placed all my more long term goals; things that perhaps will come over time. My vision board is for the things I have given priority to. It has pictures of books; I even made a picture of a book with my name on as the author. There are pictures of the band, plus text and other connected pictures. My dream book is full of pictures of things that I want to do some day, as well as places I want to visit. Whereas I look at my vision board daily, I look at my dream book on a weekly basis or when I have a quiet five minutes. I open it up and just sit back and take some time to think about the things I want out of my life.

Plus there is so much I want to do that I couldn't fit it all on a vision board and unlike my vision board, my dream book is kept out of sight but it is something I can take with me wherever I go.

Music

I don't know anyone who does not love music. Music can go along side any of our moods. If you are feeling sad or happy, chances are there is the perfect piece of music just waiting to be played. Music can also bring back happy memories from the past. I find it a great way to up lift my mood. Having joyful music in the background in a stressful situation or in a room full of negative feelings can really lighten the mood. Try it for yourself and see how it works. Music is also a great way to relax. People use music for many different reasons.

My ultimate, amazing wish, does of course involve a band. So music is a great way to help me imagine meeting them. It helps keep my mind on my wish.

The universe will work out a way to attract what it is you need and want. You are just signalling what it is you really want out of life and that you are ready to receive.

Should We Tell The World About Our Wishes?

You are doing things that can raise your energy vibrations and looking at ways to let the universe or the powers that be know exactly what it is you want out of life. Despite the fact that I had a seizure in the May, which put my first wish out of the window, I didn't let that matter. Yes, it delayed things, but I was sure the seizures would stop one day and I was convinced I was going to meet the band. I was on a high and wanted to tell the world.

But, do we tell our wishes or not? I was told when I was younger that if I told someone my wish it wouldn't come true. But was that correct? It has been said that you should keep your wishes to yourself as telling them decreases the energy of the wish. Equally, it is also said that talking to people about your wishes increases the energy.

When I first started my project I told a lot of people my wishes to increase the energy. My thought was, the more people wishing, the more energy. I learned a lesson from openly telling everyone about the book and the other things I was working towards. I thought that doing this would help raise the vibration of my wishes. Surely, I reasoned, everyone would want the best for each other? I also felt I didn't want to hide anything from my friends.

It's difficult to know what to do with so many books telling you one thing and just as many telling you another. In time I started feeling quite low about things because the responses I received were not always what I had expected. I started to feel that I was wasting my time. Yet I still had that gut feeling that I should carry on and get the book written. So that's what I did. I had learned my lesson. With those who were not so helpful, I learned to keep quiet about what I was doing and in time they forgot and got on with their lives and I got on with mine.

I don't know why some people are so negative; is it envy? Do they want a slice of what is going on in your life? Is it that they just are not connected with themselves; that they can't come up with their own ideas, so they have to take ideas from other people? I'm sure half the time people don't realize that when they are being negative they are raining on your parade. It could even be that some people are so negative about their own lives that they can't see the good in anything or in anyone else's life.

Is it harsh to say this? I know in the past I have felt the envy of others. I hope my past actions have not blocked other people's wishes and I will always be aware of this possibility when I respond to someone's ideas from now on. I'm sure a lot of people do not even realize that their thoughts and actions can be blocking your wishes.

I think telling the right people helps to give you the support you need to complete your wishes and the last thing I would want is to start keeping secrets from those close to me. True friends and the love of your family will help you along the way. They will want to see you happy; they want to help you fulfil your wishes, just as you would want the same for them. So when it comes to telling or not telling, it's up to you. Just be careful to choose wisely.

You need to remember not to let other people's opinions bring you down. It's your life you're creating and you have the possibility of making that life wonderful. Those who don't agree with what you are doing may mean well. They may want the best for you. But only you truly know what is right for yourself.

Who We Are

How you see yourself is important in terms of the law of attraction. How you feel about yourself affects your vibrations. When you feel low about yourself, your vibrations are low. When you feel good about yourself, your vibrations will be high. You attract back what you give out, like attracts like. If you want something but don't feel you are worth it, then why should you have it?

I have always been terrible at letting what other people think of me affect the way I think of myself. I used to walk into a room full of people and wonder if they liked me. Now I walk into a room, look around and wonder if I like them! You should not feel that you need to change so that other people will like you. You need to have the confidence to be yourself and trust that the right people will love you. Only change those things that you truly, in your heart, want to change, and not because of pressure from others. It's a brave person who is prepared to live and be who they truly are, without conforming to the pressure of how others expect you to be. No matter what you do in life, people will always have something to say about you. You are who you are. You are unique. You are a one off and everyone is different. Thank goodness for that and amen!

I used to wonder what people thought of me because of my memory problems. Often, I would be in mid-sentence and forget what I was talking about, or be unable to remember the name of some object. There have even been times when I just couldn't remember a person's name, even though I had known them for a long time. Usually whoever I was talking to didn't say anything, but I could tell by their facial expression that they were annoyed or found my memory lapses difficult to accept. I soon learned not to take their reaction on board. It isn't meant to be hurtful; it's down to their lack of understanding of the side effects of my epilepsy. It's important to accept that not everyone knows about epilepsy or the side effects that you may have.

Equally, there is no need to be upset if family or friends initially treat you differently. You need to remember that the diagnosis is a shock for them as well and they also need time to adjust. Remember that they mean well and do not let this period of adjustment on their part affect how you feel about yourself. It's perfectly normal for all concerned to feel stressed, upset and angry for a while. We are all human; we cannot always avoid these emotions. But you need to learn about your epilepsy together with family and friends. Together you can put things into perspective. Learn together and help each other through it.

If you are struggling to come to terms with the restrictions epilepsy has imposed on your way of life, talk to people, talk to family, friends or your doctor. There are many things you can do to adjust to the changes in your life, but whatever you do, don't give up. You need to have a positive awareness of how to approach and deal with your epilepsy. Most importantly, you have to stop it being the focal point of your life. Epilepsy is a part of you but there's a lot more to you than epilepsy.

You need to accept who you are. You may not be perfect, you may not have the perfect figure or be the perfect weight, but does it matter? You should, of course, eat a well-balanced diet and live healthily. Now, more than ever, it is important to get your five a day and get plenty of exercise. As long as you are not hurting others and are looking after yourself, does it matter what other people think? It's all about learning self-respect and loving yourself for who you are. Does it really matter if you don't have the latest gadgets, or if you don't wear clothing with a label on it, or if you have a hobby that people don't like or class as strange? Why should you allow someone else's set ideas and values to influence the way you feel about yourself and the way you enjoy your life? If everyone was identical, life would be a boring place.

It's not easy to change how you think of yourself, it doesn't happen overnight. What I did was write a list of all the things I liked about myself and every day I would remind myself of these facts, making it a habit, along with having time for myself and wearing what I like and what makes me feel good. I stopped comparing myself to others, because we are all different. I started to let the creative person in me come to the forefront. You need to find ways to promote yourself and not put yourself down. People who don't agree with your life style choices can be very hurtful with their comments but learn to ignore them. Some twenty or more years ago, when I started my paranormal investigations, I did not tell a lot of people what my hobby was. At that time interest in the paranormal was looked on as crazy and people would make fun of my involvement. Some of the things that were said were quite hurtful. Then, because of television, psychic research became the in thing to do. All of a sudden those same people who had poured scorn on my interests wanted to know me and know more about what it was I did. A part of me wanted to stand there and say, "Hold on, you used to say such and such about me, now all a sudden I'm not the freak?" But I learnt to smile and turn away. I could have said something about their past behaviour but it would have been wasted energy.

You need to accept that people are going to make comments about you no matter what you do. You are who you are and you need to love yourself for who you are. How can you expect the universe to help you with your wishes if you don't feel that you are good enough for the wishes to come true? The more positive you feel about yourself, the better your life will be and the more chance you have of fulfilling your dreams. Life is too short for you to worry what other people say or think about you. Have fun! Give them something to talk about.

You need to know that you are perfect for who you are and have faith that all your dreams will come true. You need to believe in yourself and believe that you are worth what you want out of life. You cannot change your past, but you can change and choose a wonderful future.

Remove all those restrictions you place on yourself and start to live the life you want, be the person you want to be. It's time to set yourself free and show the universe that you love yourself and that you deserve the best in life.

Remember, whatever anyone else thinks, you are more than your epilepsy and you don't have to be defined by it.

Don't Listen

There are many different kinds of gossip. There is gossip about things like celebrities and soaps. In fact there are tons of websites and magazines promoting this type of gossip. Then there is what I like to class as good gossip. This is all about the good stuff: births, marriages, what someone has achieved: that type of thing.

What I want to talk about here is what I class as harmful gossip. This is the negative gossip that goes on in the work place or between friends and family. This kind of gossip can affect us in a big way. We've probably all at one time or another been the victim of negative gossip. People make comments about you behind your back and what they've said races through your place of work or your group of friends like wild fire. By the time you hear about it, nine times out ten, the story has changed.

So why do we gossip? We all do it, I know I do. I've been right there, listening to gossip that was going on around about me, and I've returned the gossip, showing people that I was right and the other person was wrong. In my own situation all the negativity could have been avoided if the person who started the gossip had come to speak to me directly. I could have explained everything with a few words and stopped the gossip in its tracks. Equally, when I was gossiping, I could have done the right thing and gone to the person concerned directly instead of allowing myself to gossip and spread rumour around the department.

Do we do it to make ourselves feel better? Does it make us think our lives are better than whoever we are gossiping about, or, is it that we are jealous of them? When we are gossiping we often forget that the person we are talking about also has feelings. Often they do eventually get to hear what is being said about them, and that can hurt. Now we are responsible for someone getting hurt by our actions. Do you remember that old saying, 'sticks and stones may break my bones but words can never hurt me'? I think we all know that isn't true. I used to say it quite a lot when I was younger, when the bullies came towards me in the playground. It popped into my mind again when I heard people talking about me and some of the problems I have as a result of my epilepsy.

It's all too easy to fall into the negative scanning trap, focusing on what is 'wrong' with those around us. We must remember that every person is full of both loveable and loathsome traits. Try to choose to fix your gaze on all that is loveable. It's important when practicing the law of attraction to love yourself and to spread that love. By ignoring people's negative traits and getting on with your life, as well as forgiving them for saying hurtful things, you are learning to rise above the situation.

We judge others to make ourselves feel that the other person's life is going wrong while our life, of course, couldn't be better. We are so certain that the way we are is the only way to live. But stop a minute – is judging others helping you? Does it increase your vibrations and aid you in getting what you want?

Living a non-judgemental, gossip free life is not easy; in fact, could any of us manage it? I know I have mentioned this already, but no one is perfect and really do we have to be? No one has it easy and we all have our own battles to fight, all too often we don't know what people are going through. So when you get the urge, pause before judging others.

Let's stop this negative train of events, stop talking about or focusing on people's shortcoming and start to spread the sunshine: how wonderful somebody looks, what a great job they do, every time you feel a criticism coming on, substitute it with a compliment. Surely the feeling of making somebody's day by complimenting them is better than trying to put people down. This includes yourself, there is no need to brag to people how wonderful you are or try to impress them with what you have; people don't really want to hear that. But remember to have faith in yourself, feel free to give yourself a regular, well deserved, pat on the back. The words we speak or write are very powerful, they can affect people or ourselves in a positive or negative way, they can enhance our lives but they can also have the opposite effect. At the end of the day we all love compliments, so let's spread that good feeling around. Let's make people feel good about themselves and not the other way around; we have the power in ourselves to do this.

I know people reading this will have their own comments and ideas about my philosophy on life. There will be friends, family and work colleagues who will disagree with this book and there will be people I don't even know who will look at my book and think otherwise. But there will also be those who this will really resonate with and who will love and embrace my ideas whole-heartedly: those who will find what is said helpful in coping with their diagnosis and with managing their epilepsy and for me that is worth far more.

So remember that while what other people say can affect you, it also works the other way around. What you say and do can affect others and you should keep in mind that what goes around comes around. What others say and do is their karma, how you react to the situation is yours.

Out With The Old And In With The New

De-cluttering is about creating space for new things to enter our lives. Out with the old and in with the new. Have a look around your home, how much stuff do you have? Too many belongings can stop the energy flow through our homes. The less jumble we have, the more the energy can flow through. I'm sure most of you will have heard of Feng Shui. It is very much along those lines.

By de-cluttering your life you show the universe that you are ready to receive what you desire because you are making room for it. Two objects cannot occupy the same place, so by removing one object you are allowing room for something new to take its place. If, for example, you want a new car but your garage is full of clutter, what are you showing the universe? You are putting out to the universe that you don't have room for a new car; you have nowhere to keep it. By clearing the garage you are clearly signalling that you intend to manifest that new car. Perhaps you have your heart set on getting some new clothes? Clear the wardrobe out and visualise new clothing going in there. While writing this my sceptical mind did kick in; which is not a bad thing. My first thought was, if you clear your wardrobe out, you have no choice but to buy new clothes. In order for the law of attraction to work you need to believe in what you want. But I don't think it hurts to question things if you feel the need.

I thought about doing a general house clear out all in one go, but when I started there was too much I wanted to keep: all those, just in case I need, objects. So instead I'm going through my things, one at a time. I may tidy up a drawer one day then perhaps a shelf another day. Okay, it takes longer, (still an on-going thing) but by doing it this way I know that I am removing things that I won't regret later. The items that are in good condition, I send to a charity. Broken items must go, if I don't use it, I'm disposing of it. People do say 'use it or lose it'.

Once I started, I wondered why I had allowed so much stuff to accumulate. Why do we hold onto all this stuff? Does it make us feel better to feel we are keeping up with our peers? Do the items we keep make us happy? It seems that no matter how much we accumulate, we always want more. I have lost count of the amount of times I buy something; regret the purchase later and it ends up at the back of a cupboard. Reflecting on de-cluttering has helped me to save money. These days rather than just buying something because I like it, I tend to ask myself if I really need it, or is it destined to become the clutter of tomorrow? Nine times out of ten I don't buy and don't regret not having bought.

Whilst clearing out I came across so many unfinished projects, some I had never even got around to starting. I lost count of how many cross stitch kits I had still in their packets. I sold these on eBay; I looked at all the other projects and came up with a plan for finishing them. It took me a while, and slightly delayed finishing this book. I realized that by having so many unfinished projects, not only were they increasing the clutter, but the message I was sending out was that I couldn't finish what I had started and that wasn't the message I wanted to be putting out there.

Clearing out my home not only allowed the energy to flow through better, it made me feel good. Seeing space being opened up, rooms feeling bigger, being able to move around without seeing stuff piled up was a great feeling; as was knowing that I have helped others along the way by giving some of the items to charity, as well as selling some items and putting the money towards my main dream. Seeing my savings grow, knowing this was going towards the fulfilment of my ultimate, amazing wish is a wonderful high.

Take a look at your possessions with a fresh pair of eyes and ask yourself; do you love these items, do you need these items, do you use these items? If the answer is no, let them go. Don't keep them just in case they come in handy one day or because you paid a lot of money for them because they are only taking up space.

With some of the items I did not want to get rid of, mainly because there was an emotional attachment, I made space for them in cupboards so that they were not littering the lounge or bedroom. New book shelves are going into the lounge so that my books are no longer stacked high on the floor but will soon be neat. The lesson here is not just about de-cluttering, but also looking at ways in which you store things. If your home looks good and feels more open, not only will it allow a better flow of energy, just looking around the clean, clear spaces is guaranteed to lift your mood. Get rid of clutter and show the universe that you are making room for your desires to come true. You are creating a more positive environment for yourself, and removing anything that may block your dreams from manifesting.

Of course clutter isn't just about items in our homes; there is also emotional clutter, things we carry around with us all the time; things that have happened in the past or during that day, daily worries, financial or otherwise. These are all emotional clutter and these are things that we will deal with later in the book. This type of clutter is more difficult to deal with, but deal with it we must if we want to remove all the blocks from our lives and gain what it is we really want. As we clear away the jumble, both household and emotional, we are making room to attract more valuable things into our lives. Clutter is a negative thing, getting rid of negatives opens the door to positives.

Give Thanks

In July 2010 I was on top of the world, although nothing much had happened in the way of manifesting any of my dreams yet, but I knew it would happen; more importantly, it had been two and half months since my last seizure. One day I finished work and went home, walked the dogs, had something to eat, made some phone calls; I'm told I was on the phone to my younger brother when it happened. During that call I had a seizure, I don't remember making the call or anything we may have spoken about. The first thing I was aware of was being help into a chair by my husband and a friend. Slowly, it dawned on me that I had just had a seizure.

At first I got on, as I normally do, getting my life back into some kind of order. I start by getting myself moving and then I try to deal with the memory loss that always follows a seizure. At the time I didn't realize I had become very withdrawn. I felt as if everyone was against me. If I'm honest I'll admit that, at the time, I thought the law of attraction was a complete waste of time, there was no such thing. I was at an all-time low; I had reached a point where I thought the seizures would never end.

I stopped writing. Well, I thought, it doesn't work, what is the point in continuing with these dreams, it's never going to happen. I thought I was hiding what I felt quite well, until a work colleague asked me how I was, not how my health was, but how I was feeling. Apparently I had been acting odd lately. My colleague said I was snappy and that I didn't really talk to people anymore. It took just that one person asking me how I really was for me to break down and realize I wasn't coping. Having someone show me that they cared was enough for me to see there was a problem. My world was falling apart and as hard as I tried, I couldn't keep it together any more.

I took myself off to the doctor and as I sat there with her I could not speak. I was far too busy crying; crying so hard it was difficult to catch my breath. The only way I could communicate what was wrong was by writing notes. The doctor told me I was in a state of depression but because of the tablets I was on they could not give me anything to help. That was the end of the appointment: no tablets, no other help, and no helpful words.

The only thing she could do was contact my neurologist to see if the drugs I was on could be changed in case the tablets were causing the problem. I left feeling so low about life. How was I going to deal with this with no help? I walked out of the surgery feeling worse than I had when I walked in. I thought they could give me something to help lift my mood, or give me some advice on what I could do. I walked to the train station, the odd tear rolling down my cheeks. One thought kept going through my mind; how was I going to deal with this without any help? I just wanted to get home and lock the door, hide away and pretend this was not happening.

When I got home I didn't know what to do; all I was certain of was that I couldn't carry on like this. In that moment, I had the strongest urge to carry on with my project. With no idea which way to go, I picked up the phone, called my parents and best friend and admitted I wasn't coping. I admitted I had depression. Just admitting it to people, admitting that I was not coping, was like a major weight being lifted off me. I was learning that accepting help makes me no lesser a person. I finally accepted I had epilepsy and there was nothing I could do to fight it. That evening I thought of ways that I might be able to help myself and I looked to the law of attraction for help. I wrote a list of all the things I hated about my life and burnt it. I thought that would make me feel better but it didn't. Then I wrote a list of all the things I wanted out of life, thinking that seeing the things I wanted would help, but it didn't. Finally, I wrote a list of all the things I was grateful for in my life. Seeing that list, things like my family, my home, my job, made me feel so much better about myself. Although I was feeling negative about the epilepsy there was so much in my life that I was thankful for and that lifted my spirits. I looked at my list every night, and before I knew it, I had started to feel better about life. After a while I started to feel great about myself, and in time I could see a way forward again. I didn't put any pressure on myself, I allowed myself time to heal.

By the time I saw the neurologist I was feeling much better about myself. We discussed it and agreed that it wasn't the tablets that were causing the depression so there was no need to change my medication. He did increase the amount I was on though, as we both agreed that the last seizure was the cause of my depression. I had just had enough and I admitted that after it happened I felt as if they were never going to stop.

By giving thanks I saw what a wonderful group of people I have around me. I'm not saying that the law of attraction helped to stop the seizures, but so far it has helped me to deal with my epilepsy. It turned out that the seizure in July 2010 was in fact my last ever seizure, the seizure that really broke me. Is it possible that you have to hit rock bottom before things start to change in your life? Perhaps that isn't the case but it seemed like it to me, because after that seizure and the depression that followed I have never looked back.

Something as simple as giving thanks for all that I have, really, really, worked in such a big way. It helped relieve the depression without having any tablets do the job for me. I managed to shake of its grip and that gave me such a buzz.

No matter what we do in life everyone is going to go through periods of feeling low, negative and angry. Instead of panicking and analysing we should aim more for acceptance. Very few people, no matter how happy they seem, will escape those feelings totally. What we have to remember is that these low periods are going to pass and our happy feelings will return. When they do, give thanks for the happy times, it will make you feel so much better.

Whether you do or don't like the idea of the law of attraction, at the end of each day, give thanks for all the good things that have happened that day, give thanks for what is in your life. Say your thanks out loud or start a journal. It's a great mood lifter because not only are you showing the universe how thankful you are for all the good times and the great people, it will also bring home to you what is good in your life. This raises your vibration and will attract more good things into your life. Like attracts like.

Something that also gave me a major boost during my time of depression was being able to successfully face one of my major fears: talking in public. My brother was getting married in the August and he asked me to be his best woman. It was such a great pleasure to be asked, until I realized I would have to give a speech in front of a lot of people, most of whom I didn't know. I couldn't talk about facing your fears if I couldn't show that I could face mine. So I faced it head on and gave the speech. Although I was somewhat nervous I did it and people even laughed in the right places. I came out of it alive. Facing my anxiety left me feeling amazing.

Then, in the September, something happened which made me realize my ultimate, amazing wish could in fact really materialize. The band announced they had a name for their new album. That was all; no release date or what would be happening after the album was released. But, don't ask me how, I just knew this was the turning point and that kicked me back into my project. I became convinced that I really was going to meet the band. The news of their album made me truly believe my dreams were going to come true and I gave thanks for this. The news had come at just the right time. It gave me the boost I needed to continue on with the project. I could see a light at the end of the tunnel and I haven't looked back since.

Take Time Out To Relax

By the time the album name was released I was starting to feel better about myself and I felt that the depression had almost gone. I still had the odd bad day, but then, don't we all? I still wasn't writing, I thought it was important to get myself together before I carried on with anything else. I was beginning to think about re-starting my writing and carrying on with my project but I couldn't decide where to start. Then, one day, I was reading about relaxing and taking time out sounded like a good reason to have an afternoon nap. I turned on the TV and lay on the sofa and closed my eyes. Then something strange happened.

I knew I had been asleep, but what happened next felt so real, so much so I'm not sure if I dreamt it or if it really happened.

I woke up with a fright, the room was darker than it should have been, but standing by the sofa I could see a person, although I couldn't make out who it was. I could see their hands, clasped together, then their hands opened up to look like a book. It was the type of thing you would do if you were playing charades. I lay there, staring at this person. It felt like a long time but it could only have been a matter of minutes, if that. Then the person disappeared and the room became lighter. I couldn't quite believe what I had just seen.

I got up and made myself a coffee, still trying to get my head around what had just happened. I had this strong urge deep inside that I had to finish the book. This little voice in my head was saying: it's time to stop moping around; it's time to get back to it. To this day, I don't know with any certainty what happened, whether it was real or a dream, but I was certain I had to carry on. So, coffee in hand, I got all my notes out and started to re-read them.

Our lives are so busy, work, family, the home, the list just seems to go on and we forget to take time out to relax. But it doesn't help our stress levels to be on the go all the time, constantly worrying about what is going on around us. Stress can cause many health problems and taking just a few minutes each day, longer if at all possible, can help. Relaxing is a great way to clear our heads from everyday worries.

I may not always have shown it, but I used to worry a lot. I worried about how other people saw me and about how my life was going. If I had a disagreement with someone I would find myself worrying about that, and then I wouldn't sleep that night. The less slumber I got, the more worried I would be. There were too many nights when my mind was going ten to the dozen and I couldn't drop off for worrying.

My neurologist kept asking me if I was getting enough sleep as a lot of seizures were happening during the time I was starting to wake up. Of course I didn't admit the truth, at the time I was still pretending I was dealing with everything. I could not admit that some nights I was too scared to sleep in case I woke up to having a seizure. I understood the lack of rest wasn't helping, but you can't force yourself to sleep. He must have sensed something though, as he suggested I try listening to music as I lay in bed as it might help me to relax. It worked wonders and it's something I still do now if I'm having one of those nights when my mind is all over the place.

We need our slumber; we need to relax, not just for our minds but for our health. As I started to do this more I had a much clearer head about things and my sleep improved. When I had a bad day at work or what people were saying started getting on top of me, at the end of the day, I would come home and have a shower. I would imagine all those negative thoughts and negative events being washed away from me. The only thing that would be left was positive thought.

If I'm still thinking about things by the time I go to bed another thing that I find really works is to slow my breathing down. As I breathe in I imagine I breathe in white, positive light and I breathe out black, negative light. After a while the black light becomes grey, and then white, as all the negative stuff has left my body. I can't remember where I got this from but it really does work to help me relax my mind, ready for a better night's rest.

There are so many aids to relaxation: meditation, yoga, or simply having a hot bath, listening to music, walking the dog. All are great ways to shut the world out and just relax. Each of us has to find their own way to unwind, these are only ideas. It doesn't always have to be for long, 15 minutes a day is enough for some people. Find what works best for you and take regular time out for yourself. This just may help your life to be less stressful and will improve your health and well-being.

Relaxing isn't just about taking time out, it's also about looking around and seeing what is causing the stress. Why are you getting stressed about situations that are perhaps out of your control? This is something we will come back to later, but for now, try going with the flow of life instead of trying to go against it or control it. Life, after all, is to be enjoyed.

Unwinding and taking time out not only helps you with other areas of the law of attraction, it also helps you to have faith. Faith is so important, we need to believe that what we want will come to us and that we deserve to reach our goals in life. We need that belief to keep us going, to motivate us to strive for what we want and show the universe that we believe in our wishes and that they are right for us. Without that belief we have nothing to work on to show the universe it is really this we want. If we don't feel that we deserve our wishes why will the universe help us to achieve them?

I firmly believed I would meet the band by the end of the project; something inside me reinforced that feeling. So imagine my joy when that November the first single was released, followed by the album. But more importantly, the tour dates were given out. Oh yes, we had dates! In the following May/June they would be touring; slightly out of my project time, but who's keeping tabs.

When I started this, I don't think I really thought it was going to happen. At the time I only knew that they were going back to the studio to start on a new album. Yet here I was, new album in hand, tour just around the corner, a perfect way to end the project and a wonderful way to finish the book. Meeting the band would prove to me that the law of attraction works. I had a feeling inside that everything would turn out just fine.

We need to learn to calm the mind and learn patience; not everything we want is going to come to us right this second. Things do take time, so take time out and relax. We can't control what happens in life so there is no real reason for us to get so stressed about it.

I do firmly believe that everything we need will come to us at the right time.

Say It As You Believe

Okay. I'm going to be honest, when I started to look at affirmations I could not bring myself to stand in front of the mirror in the morning saying things like, "I'm wonderful," and thankfully we don't have to. Because every thought we have, every word we say is an affirmation. Remember, like attracts like, and this also applies to how we think about ourselves. Saying things like, "I'm not good enough," is a negative affirmation. Instead, use a positive affirmation, saying something like, "I'm lucky in everything." Saying and believing positive things goes back to how we feel about ourselves.

Affirmations are short, positive statements and I have found them a good way to start the day because they help me to get into a positive mind-set. Ideally you should begin each day with a positive spirit and full of enthusiasm because who knows what wonderful things that day is going to bring you. Remember, life is to be enjoyed, you only have one life so make the most of it and get out there and enjoy it.

Have you ever heard yourself saying, "I got out of bed on the wrong side today"? I have, normally when I'm having a bad day. That would shortly be followed by my saying, "Everything that could go wrong is." I would normally say this when I was in a bad mood and easily annoyed, as if saying it made me feel better that I had just shouted at someone. But is this really how we want to start our day – on a negative, because how we begin our day can make or break it. Our initial attitude and actions have a strong effect on the rest of the day. Waking up and thinking that we got out of the wrong side of the bed will only encourage negative things to happening to us because that is the mind-set we are already in.

We need to start our day on a positive note, in a positive mind-set, fully expecting that today is going to be a wonderful day. So in the mornings, when I look outside, with my coffee in my hand, I say, "Today is going to be a wonderful day" or "Everything is going to be okay." That gives me a great feeling to start my day with.

When my depression started, although giving thanks for all that I had really helped, there were times during the day when I needed a little lift. When this happened I would take a couple of deep breaths and say something positive like, "Life really is wonderful."

Before the depression, and for years, I thought I wasn't good enough to have what I wanted and then I became a qualified practitioner and I started to change my way of thinking. After a while though, those old feeling started again. I had always wanted to write a book and would often have ideas, but again, I didn't think I was good enough. I thought I could never be lucky enough to meet the band, or I couldn't progress in my career because my face didn't fit. I had fallen back into the negative trap. All my thoughts, everything I was saying was a negative affirmation of my life and I was doing it without realizing.

Then I developed epilepsy and discovered the law of attraction and my views, in time, started to change. When I first started saying affirmations, honestly, I felt silly. Part of me thought that it was a silly subject and I couldn't really believe what I was saying. It was during the period of the depression that I really got to grips with using affirmations because they really helped, they helped to lift my mood when I was really down. Affirmations can help you change the way you feel about yourself. Deep down you need to believe you are worthwhile and deserving of having all the things you want out of life and affirmations can help.

Living in a positive way is not always easy. We all go through low periods. When things are getting to you, you need to remember that life is too short to be anything but happy. Being low is a part of life, getting yourself back up is living. Never give up, life is out there for you to go and get.

When you are having a low period, you need to be aware of your affirmations. It is important not to let too many negative thoughts become affirmations. If you have a negative thought don't worry about it, forgive yourself. Don't waste energy focusing on negativity. If you put energy into these thoughts it is the same as giving your energy to positive thought. Just shrug the negative thought away and carry on with your day. Let's face it, we all have bad days. You can't control day to day eventualities, but you can shape your future.

You might even decide to change your negative thought into something positive. 'I'm not that lucky' can, with just a little effort, instead become 'of course I'm lucky, I'm lucky because I have —' add something that you feel lucky about. This way you're giving thanks and affirming that you are lucky because you have something in your life that you are thankful about.

Some affirmations will feel natural. Say them with passion. The higher your emotional state as you say them, the more effective they are. If you want to construct your own, choose your words carefully. Words are powerful things. Words like should, could or might are out. Instead of saying, "I could be lucky" say "I'm lucky." Saying, "I am" rather than, "I could be" carries far more power.

The ones I like at the moment are: 'I am happy, healthy and wealthy', 'I act on my inspirations', 'I'm filled with creative energy', and, 'I'm always happy, respected and in need of nothing'. You can construct your own, or, have a look around the Internet for ideas; include your wishes if you want to. You don't have to use the same ones, change them whenever you like. My feeling is that if you keep using the same ones, it becomes routine and there is a chance you might lose the emotion behind the saying and keeping that emotional content high is so important.

And yes I feel it does work, because look at me now, doing something I never thought I was good enough to do: writing this book.

Things Start To Change

It's the start of 2011 and my excitement is running high. We had just bought our eight concert tickets and we were extra organised and had also booked our hotel rooms. The only thing that remained between now and the concerts was to decide what to wear. That would take a lot of thought and planning; after all I was going to meet the band.

I was so focused on the up and coming tour and working on my book that I realized I had stopped counting time since my last seizure, yet the fear of having another one was still there. Like a lot of people with epilepsy, I count time in between seizures, to see if there's a pattern. I also count time between them to see if they are stopping: are they becoming less frequent, are they coming to an end? I don't know at what point I thought about the seizures but I saw that it had been six months since my last one, and, if I continued seizure free, in another six months, I could get my driving licence back.

With this realization I started to feel really nervous about them starting up again now that I was so close to getting my diving licence back. I needed something to take my mind off the possibility. Then, one day, I was reading a magazine and saw an advert for a course. This would give me something to focus on and would be a big boost to my confidence.

The advert was for a weekend course in London, during February. The course was being run by an author from America and I had read some of her books with a great deal of interest. As soon as I saw the advert I had a strong urge to go but I put it off for a few days. I tried to talk myself out of it. I started to let the old fears back in: the thought of being with a group of strangers for a whole weekend, the thought of having a seizure when I was alone and in a place I hardly knew.

I couldn't stop thinking about the course though, so I took a deep breath and sent them an email to see if there was still a space free. In the back of my mind I thought it was already too late, but, if I was meant to go, there would be a place. There was in fact one place left, so I booked it.

Now I really had to deal with any fear I had of having a seizure. I also had to find the strength to be away with a bunch of strangers, and in London, somewhere I don't go too often. So with everything booked, off I went to London. I had the most amazing time, met some lovely people, got around London on my own without getting lost, and the course was really interesting and gave me a lot to think about.

When it came to leaving, I was feeling very positive about life. If I could do this, I could do anything. I started to really think about the future. By the time I arrive back home from the course it had been seven months since my last seizure.

Life Is Now

Wonderful or not, the past has been and gone. You can't stay in the past forever. There is nothing, absolutely nothing you can do to change it. So is there any point replaying the events in your mind over and over again? Surely by doing this you are living in the past and allowing it to bring you down emotionally? You are therefore damaging yourself. How can you move forward if you are still stuck in the past? What if you're missing great opportunities today because you are too busy thinking about what has already gone? The past is past.

Your past has helped to make you who you are but you can't let your past decide your future. I know that it isn't always easy but you have to learn to live in the now and look forward to the future. Too often I hear people say that they can't do things or go places because of a past event. Or they do things because of something that happened in the past. But is it right to live that way? Or is it making an event from the past into a fear of today? Are you allowing your past to stop you from enjoying today, and the rest of your future?

Whatever has happened cannot be changed so why spend your time thinking about it and re-playing it over and over? It doesn't help anyone, least of all you. Think what you could be missing today because you're so busy thinking of your past. Every day is another chance to change your life; you are never too young or too old to change what you want and where you are going. This also applies to past regrets: for things done and things you didn't do. You have to learn to stop saying, "I wish I had done —" Move your regrets, put them on your to do list.

Remember, it makes you no lesser a person to ask for help to understand and overcome things. If anything, it shows that you are stronger because you are prepared to face what has happened and prepared to take what can be a hard journey to overcome past trauma. You are drawing a line and not letting your past stop you from doing what you want in the future. Life is to be enjoyed.

It's not just about your past but every day. Perhaps someone has a disagreement with you, forgive them. You don't know what has led them to that moment. Is the disagreement going to change your life, or is it better to walk away? We have to remember that each new day will soon be a yesterday. I'm not encouraging you to count time away, but don't allow other people's problems to become your own, go out there and enjoy life.

Just as important as not getting stuck in the past, spending too much time thinking of your future is also detrimental. Spending all your time dwelling on what you want to materialize can lead to you missing out on enjoyment of what you have now. The future is your motivation, it's your dreams, it's what you are working towards. But this should not mean spending so much time working hard towards what you want that you end up losing sight of today. It can be hard to balance your career, the house, the kids, the list is endless, but don't miss the opportunity right in front of you, those special moments that will become the happy memories of your future. Don't put too much pressure on yourself in your determination to work everything out.

I'm not saying you should not make some plans, or work towards something, I found it useful to have a plan because it helped me to keep focused, but you should not let this take all your time up or let your future plans take all your focus. Remember each day is a new day and it's out there for you to live, to enjoy, to have fun. Enjoy life for what it is today because who knows what other wonders there are in store for you tomorrow.

As I write these words, I have a week off work. In my mind I wanted to spend as much time as possible in finishing this book. So much so that when a friend asked me out to lunch my first instinct was to put her off. I was getting so stressed out about getting things done. My book, like a lot of things I'm doing, is for my future. But I let myself forget to live in the now. I enjoy writing but there is no point working my fingers to the bone during a week off work without taking time out to enjoy my life.

I have been surprised by how many people drag themselves around each day. Instead of appreciating each and every moment they dwell on problems and unhappiness. This doesn't achieve anything, apart from making you miserable. Is that how you want to live your life? Are you going to spend your days worrying about what could happen: worrying about what others think? It's not easy when you have epilepsy not to worry about when the next seizure is going to be, or how other people see you but in order to enjoy the life you have now it is necessary to try to rise above a habitual pattern of negative fears. I know it's not easy but you have to let go of your fear and see what is out there for you.

Don't sit at home worrying, be out there, enjoying your life, ignore what others may be thinking about you. It is your life; how you live it is up to you. As long as you are not hurting people or breaking the law, does it matter what others may think. As I have said before, we are all different, if we all liked and enjoyed the same things life would be boring. Remember also that this applies to everyone else; accept that they may be different to you and like different things; encourage them in doing what they enjoy.

We live in a wonderful world. Life is always on the move, nothing stays the same, there will always be sadness and life may not seem fair at times. Living in a positive mind-set may not stop problems occurring, or solve them when they do. But a positive mind-set will help you to see problems in a different light and can make solving them a more pleasant experience. You have to accept that things don't always happen the way you want them to, but when that happens, just wonder to yourself if there is a reason for this, then, let the thought go. Don't waste time worrying about it.

Of course you do need to take other people's feelings into account but if those people love you then they won't stop you doing what you want to do or being who you want to be, they will support you and help you if they can; just as we should aim to do for them.

So, the past was a lesson, the future is your goal, your motivation. The now is for living, for having fun, for enjoying your life, enjoying the life that you want. Enjoy every moment because who really knows what's going to happen in the future.

Laughter

We all like to have a good laugh, but do we do it enough? Laughter is such a positive thing; it generates positive energy, opens your heart and elevates your vibrations.

If you're feeling low having a good laugh releases feel good hormones which lift your mood. Have you ever been feeling low and heard people laughing and, without there being any other reason, your mood has suddenly lifted? There has been extensive research into laughter being good for us and helping to relieve stress, as well as being beneficial to our health and our moods. It's that old saying 'laughter is the best medicine'. Laughter can help to restore a positive mind-set. It can also bring people together and help us to connect. Laugh often, even when you don't feel like it, laughing will make you feel so much better. Sometimes we are all so busy getting on with our daily chores that I think we forget to live in the now and enjoy life and have a good laugh with friends and family. There's no harm if right now you don't feel that you're in a place where you feel like laughing. Try surrounding yourself with positive people; you'll be surprised how their mood can quickly rub off onto you.

We also need to smile more often; you don't feel like smiling right now? Think of something funny and feel that smile happen. I love it when I'm in a crowded room and I start to smile and all of sudden people want to know what I'm smiling about. A simple smile can lift a mood no end.

Spend time with people you care about, or in doing activities that you enjoy. These are the things that will make you happy; these will give you something to smile about. Laugh and watch how that laughter rubs off onto others. See for yourself, have a good laugh about something and see the mood it gives you. It's hard to feel angry, disheartened or guilty and humours at the same time.

Enjoy life, stop worrying about things you can't change, let your inner child out and have a good laugh. Try doing childish things every now and then. If you're out for a walk with family, run ahead and leap out at them from behind a tree. Try anything that will lighten the mood. Find out what it is that makes you laugh, let your hair down.

Forgiveness

Forgiveness is a difficult subject to cover but one we need to address in order to carry on with positive living. Forgiveness is a decision to let go of bitterness and resentment towards another person or situation. Bitterness or anger is such a negative thing, plus by not forgiving, we continue to live in the past. In letting go of this negativity we are removing the focus and attention from these unwanted feelings and we can let positive energy replace them.

Learning to forgive ourselves is sometimes easier than forgiving things that have happened to us in the past but unless we can forgive and carry on, the negative feelings will build up and may result in anger and lead to using those past experiences to avoid similar situations in an attempt to prevent getting hurt again. Holding onto past trauma inevitably results in being negative and possibly in feeling that you don't deserve good things; you don't deserve to have your dreams come true.

Once you forgive you will experience a sense of relief. Carrying around all that negativity is like carrying around a large weight. Forgive the past and that weight will go leaving you free to move onto much better things. The negative feelings that you carry towards those who have hurt you will not bring justice, they really only affect you. Those who hurt you will have their own karma to deal with, as the saying goes, 'what goes around comes around'.

Nobody is perfect, we all make mistakes. The bitterness and anger you may feel towards someone will not affect them in the way you might wish. They may or may not know that they have upset you. If they are aware that they have hurt you then show that you have risen above it by living a successful and happy life.

Be strong enough to forgive rather than fight. Bear in mind that you don't know what has led them to this point. Don't let what has happened ruin your day, don't let it stop you from enjoying your life.

Sometimes it is hard to forgive but try looking at the events again and see if anything positive can come out of it. Look at ways you can use what happened, perhaps to help other people who are going through the same thing. Working with your past experience can be painful to start with but think of the people you're helping, you're showing them that there is a light at the end of the tunnel. By giving others hope you will also be helping yourself by turning a negative situation into a positive one.

Forgive those people who look at you oddly when you tell them you have epilepsy. Often people who act differently towards you when they find out just don't understand. Try to remember that all some people know about this illness is what they have read. No one can really know what it's like unless they have experienced it at first hand. What you can do is to fight back against lack of knowledge in a positive way by raising awareness. Be prepared to talk about epilepsy and educate people, enabling them to know what it is like. In this way, one day, people will begin to understand more about what those who have this condition are going through.

It isn't just about forgiving others though: we also need to forgive ourselves. I had to forgive myself for not talking more about my illness. Perhaps if I had been more open about how I felt, the depression would never have happened. But it did and I've had to forgive myself for that. Over the last few months I've learned a lot about myself and my coping mechanisms, the most important part was the realization that I needed to be more open with my family and friends about how I was feeling. So, please don't hide, talk to people about what you are going through and how you are dealing with it. Those who are close to you do want to help; you just have to let them.

Perhaps the single biggest act of forgiveness I had to accomplish was to be able to forgive the illness itself. Achieving this helped me conquer my depression because, although I had accepted that I now had this condition, I needed to go through a process of forgiving it: forgiving it for how it changed my life in such a short period of time. I began by starting a list of all the things I thought were negative and then all the positive things that had come about since the first seizure. At first this was hard but then I really thought about all I had done since then and perhaps wouldn't have done if it hadn't been for the epilepsy.

One of the most positive things to come out of it all was that it showed me what a wonderful group of people I have around me, giving me their support. Nor would I have started this journey if it hadn't been for my illness, I would never have found the courage to write this book. Epilepsy has perhaps given me more to look forward to in life than I would have had if I had never been diagnosed.

When I was first diagnosed I would never have believed that I would ever see epilepsy in a positive light, but here I am on this amazing journey of self-discovery and I'm loving every minute of it. Life does not thrive on regrets or anger stemming from the past. Life is the here and now, enjoy the life you have.

None of us are perfect, we all make mistakes but it's how we deal with those mistakes that is important. We need to forgive ourselves and others because holding onto the past is a negative thing. Remember, when you fall off your positive perch, you need to forgive yourself. Don't beat yourself up about it; it happens to all of us.

Random Acts Of Kindness

Just when I thought life could not get any better, it did. Something amazing happened, something that I never thought possible.

You know what it's like when you're watching television and you see a show and wish you were there, taking part. You may say to yourself, "Aren't they lucky. That would never happen to me." I've done this in the past, sat wishing I was there and thinking I'm just not that lucky. Well that was soon to change because it turned out I was that lucky person, well one of many, but that's not the point. For the first time in my life I had the chance to be involved in something extraordinary, something I would never have believed would happen to me.

The band was doing a one off TV show in the March. Tickets were limited and although my friend and I were up early the day the tickets went on sale, we were not lucky enough to get any. We were, however, put on the reserved list. The only problem with that was we might not know until the day whether or not we would get in. So putting caution to one side, we planned to go to London on the day in the hope that we would get in to see the show. Then one person's act of kindness changed the situation. The person had managed to acquire too many tickets and had posted on a social network to see if anyone wanted them. Incredibly, no one else replied except us.

On the day my excitement was sky high. I just could not believe how lucky I was and all thanks to someone's act of kindness. That act of kindness was going to allow me to attend an event I never thought I would be lucky enough to be part of. The night was amazing, out of this world, and I was on an almighty high. Things were getting better and better almost by the day.

It got me thinking. What did I do to make others people's days? The answer that came back was not one I was very happy with. I'm not talking just about the big stuff, like the act of kindness that a complete stranger had just done for me, but the small everyday kindnesses everyone can easily do. Sometime the smallest act of kindness is worth more than the grandest intention.

A random act of kindness is a selfless act that we freely give because we want someone to be happy, without expecting anything in return. Doing something nice for someone else is its own reward. Carrying out such an act will of itself improve your feeling of wellbeing and happiness.

It's an amazing thing that each of us has the power to brighten someone's day by doing a simple act of kindness. It can be whatever you want it to be, small or big, it doesn't matter. What matters is that the action comes from your heart. What you do doesn't have to cost much or indeed, anything at all. It's just a way to show someone you care, that you've been thinking about them. It could be as simple as opening the door for someone, speaking kindly, or praising someone's efforts. Anything at all that might put a smile on someone's face or make a positive difference in their day. Opportunities to do something random are available for you to take up at any time, every day and anywhere.

The other day I went shopping and had quite a lot in my trolley. Whilst standing in the queue, I noticed the gentleman behind me only had a few items so I asked him if he would like to go before me as I had quite a lot. He was shocked; no one had ever done such a thing for him before. This small act of kindness, he said, had made his day. Is this the world you want to live in; a place where people are shocked that a stranger can do something nice for them?

Try it for yourself, see the smile on someone's face and know that you are responsible for putting it there. Enjoy the amazing feeling you get from doing something nice. Performing even the smallest act of kindness will give you a boost; it will make you feel good about yourself and leave you with such a positive feeling. Even if you are feeling low, doing something to help someone else will leave you with a big smile on your own face.

The more I do, the more I want to do. Seeing that I can make someone's day makes me feel good. My view on acts of kindness is that, kindness is not an act, it's a lifestyle. Let's get out there and help others, whether human, animal, wildlife or nature. Some people give up their spare time to do some amazing things for charity; others do what they can to help our wildlife and the land. Doing what feels right in your heart shows the universe that you are willing to share all that you have, whether it's time or money. A random act of kindness and giving is showing love, it's also showing that you are ready to receive, plus it makes you feel good. Everyone has something to contribute, just do what your heart tells you is right. Let's make this world a better place for all of us to live in.

This Earth has a lot to offer us; from our everyday needs like food and water to our education and entertainment. We can take and take, but should we keep taking if we don't put something back?

'Give to receive' is an old saying, but should we give and expect things in return? Like attracts like. If you want kindness, be kind. If you want love, be loving. What you give out you will receive. But you have to give to receive. Give for the joy of giving, give freely and cheerfully, give from the heart. If you want more love, give love. If you want more respect give respect. Whatever you want out of life, give it away first.

Doing things because you feel like you have to isn't as powerful as truly giving from the heart. Whatever energy you give out will be returned. Doing good deeds raises our vibrations and makes us happier. It doesn't matter what we give, we all have something to contribute, time, money, talent, knowledge. It doesn't have to be about giving money, it can be as simple as sharing a book.

I love giving gifts, more so if they are made by me and even better if they are unexpected. It always puts a smile on the receiver's face and often marks the person's day as special. Money can be tight at times, so if I can't give a lot of money, I always put my change in the charity boxes that are usually by the cash till.

I would like to point out that doing random acts of kindness doesn't mean you should become a doormat or exhaust yourself. We know that there are a minority of people who will just keep taking. The problem is this kind of behaviour causes you to start grudging what you give and that is not the message you want to send out.

Giving is not just about giving to others; it's also about giving to yourself. There is no point giving to others if you don't also look after yourselves. Giving to others makes us feel good about ourselves but giving to ourselves makes us feel good too. Your gift to yourself can be a simple five minutes of time set aside for peace and quiet.

Just as giving is important, learning to receive is also important. I used to shy away from praise and found it difficult to receive gifts. The message I was unconsciously sending out, of course, was that I wasn't ready to receive any of my wishes. I had to learn to change my mental attitude. I had to realize that along with sending out my negative message to all and sundry, I was also depriving the giver of their full measure of joy in being able to give.

You deserve to receive. You work hard; you do all you can to help others, so why shouldn't you receive? When you give you should not expect to receive straight away. It may not be in the next hour, or even within the next week. But you will receive and you must keep faith in that.

The more you live this way, the more natural it will be and soon you will become a naturally giving person, it will be part of your nature. Giving and receiving is fun and can bring great contentment into your life, whether you choose to live life by the law of attraction or not. If we all lived this way we could make the world a better place.

Stop

We seem to live in a world where people constantly complain. The next time you're out and about just take a few minutes to listen. Here are some of the complaints I heard the last time I carried out this experiment

- Not having enough time.
- The weather is bad, it's too cold, it's too hot.
- Work.
- Road closures.
- Train running late.

Complaining about things you can't change and have no control over doesn't make you feel any better. In fact it can bring you down, as well as those around you, because you are focusing on the negative things in your life instead of focusing your energy on the positives.

By complaining all you do is show the universe that your life is not perfect, so in theory, that is what you attract to yourself: imperfection. I'm terrible at complaining. I complain that I have so much I want to do and not enough time to do it. If I saved the time that I use up complaining, I would have the time I need to complete all the things on my to-do list.

Someone at work complained about me once. At the time I was shocked, but stepping back from the situation I soon realized, really, what did I expect. I was so busy complaining that I was bound to annoy someone into making a complaint about me.

Why is it that we want to talk about the bad things rather than focusing on the good? It doesn't make us feel better, but we all do it. Instead, try focusing on the good. Let your mind be filled with times someone does a good job rather than thinking about when they do a bad one.

A little while ago I stayed at a hotel. The staff were so helpful that I wrote a letter to tell the manager. I got a nice reply, thanking me for my comments. He also made sure the staff on duty saw the letter. It gave me a nice feeling to know I might have brightened their day. It's horrible if all you hear all day is complaint after complaint, or how you could do better. We could all make a difference by telling people when they do a good job. Those small words can make a big difference to how someone feels about themselves. They may even try harder because they know they are valued.

Bottom line: stop complaining, focus on the good things about a person and what they do; focus on the good things in your life, the good things that are happening around you, rather than the not so good.

When someone asks you how you are, don't say, "Yeah, I'm okay" instead say, "I'm great thanks" or "Isn't it a lovely day." Compliment rather than complain, appreciate rather than criticize, look for the good not the bad. A different mind set can change the way you feel about yourself and those around you.

Words are powerful, what we say and how we say it can change our own or someone else's day. Focusing on the bad is negative, focusing on the good is positive and we want to attract more of the positive into our lives.

Choices

We all have choice; we choose how to live our lives. The choices that you make today sculpt your lives in the future, which is why it's so important to live in the now, because the decisions you make now lead you closer or further away from your goals.

The process of choice is a mental process of judging the merits of multiple options and selecting one; the option that feels right to you. Nobody can tell you which choice to make; nobody can tell you what to do. They may offer advice but it is your decision alone; it's your life, you are the one living it, the responsibility is yours.

Every day there are a series of choices: what to wear, which way you will travel to work, mundane decisions which have to be made. But there are other selections you undertake that lead to your destiny. You make choices about all your actions in life, such as how you treat others, how you communicate with others and how you can help or hurt others. You pick the kind of job that you want to do, where you want to live, and the kind of families that you want to have. If you select the things you love then you will attract the things you love. It also means that if you choose the things you don't like, then you will attract more of the things you hate. Working with the law of attraction is not about if you are lucky or not. A lot of how your life is now is a result of the decisions you have made. Pick the things that make you feel good rather than those that make you feel bad. Like attracts like.

Is there such a thing as a wrong choice? At the time you may have felt you were selecting the right option but it hasn't turned out the way you hoped. Making a different decision back then is no guarantee that things would have turned out any better. It could be that the alternative would have made your life much worse than it is now. Whatever the result might have been, that option is now in the past and it is pointless thinking about it as you can't go back in time to change the decision you made.

Whatever choice you made in the past, if it is negatively impacting on your life now, you still have the ability to make a different choice. Nothing is set in stone. You can either sit around and accept what life has thrown at you or you can stand tall and leave no room for doubt that you want your dreams and goals and are prepared to go out there and get them.

When you make a decision you need to follow your heart. Do what feels right for you. Let any major choices come from your heart, not from your ego. Living from your heart will make your life a lot happier. You are the author of your life, if you want to change something then only you can do so.

Of course what you decide can affect your friends, your families, your co-workers, and anybody else that comes into your life. This can sometimes make it hard to know what to do and there will be times when it's a family decision not just your own, like where to live, where to go on holiday. But what you enjoy doing or where life may be taking you, your hobbies, what you believe in, is up to you. These are just examples but I'm sure you get the idea. There are some choices that need to be made as a family and then there are others you are free to make on your own. Whatever or however you make your choices, do it from the heart.

Each day we can go to work the normal way or take a different route; do you turn left or right? Do you stop at that shop or not? The list is never ending. People with epilepsy (in fact those with any illness) have the choice to either let the condition control them or not. For a while I did, I wouldn't go places because of taking my tablets and because of the fear of seizures. I was so worried that I would forget things that the routine I began putting in place because of memory loss was getting in the way of me living my life. I made the decision that I would no longer allow epilepsy to control my life. Nor would I continue to fit my life around it. Yes, epilepsy is a part of my life but now it no longer controls me.

The first thing I did was to buy one of those trays in which you can store your medication, with the days of the week and the times when to take the medication marked on. Each Sunday I arrange my medication and take my tablets with me each day. I'm no longer going to be subjected to missing things because of epilepsy and the need to remember my tablets. It's now part of my daily routine, a routine that helps me not to forget these important things. I have a diary that I use for everyday things, even down to what I may need to pick up from the shops. I do anything I can to make my life run more smoothly. And it works; I'm able to more freely attend last minute events without having to worry about things like tablets. Mobile phones are great; I set alarms and reminders on mine, so I know I'll never forget important things, such as my medication.

It may be a small thing, but some small decisions can have a big impact on your life. I choose to live, I choose to live the life I want and epilepsy is not going to stop me. There will be people out there who won't believe in the law of attraction; there may be people who will think the whole idea is crazy, but that is their choice, it isn't for anyone else to judge them and their beliefs. We are all free to believe in whatever we wish. Otherwise the world would be a harsh place indeed.

People will judge me for my ideas and all that I plan to do in the future. I'm sure you will find the same thing, but you have to ignore them, it's their choice to be judgemental, you don't need to repay their judgement. The law of attraction will do that for you. You can listen to people telling you how to live your life and still carry on with your own path. Let your path include living without judgement of others, take care of your own world. You can think for yourself, no matter what anyone else has to say.

The law of attraction has given me hope. Hope that I can achieve whatever my heart desires. This isn't selfish, this is taking responsibility for my life; this is me allowing myself to be happy. There is nothing wrong with being grateful and thankful for all that I have and for all that is coming to me. This is my choice, to seize the moment and enjoy life. Let today be the first day of your new and exciting life.

The Project To Date

A Quick Update Of Things So Far

One of the best things about keeping a journal of your journey is being able to see things unfold in front of you. I know I have a memory problem but it has been interesting to read back in my journal and have that sudden thought of 'oh my, I remember that', about something that I had forgotten. It's also a reminder that there are wonderful things that happen to us, but there are also not so good things that happen every now and then.

Going back to my main wish, everything seemed to be happening so fast, but I finally felt that everything was coming together. Life was full of ups and downs. I was behind on writing this book; too busy listening to what people had to say about the band touring and how crazy I was for doing all that I had planned. But it was my choice and I was going to do it no matter what anyone else had to say. This book was going to be published and I was going to meet the band.

I couldn't believe where time had gone. It wasn't all that long ago I was counting the weeks till the tour. I still had no idea how I was going to meet them, or when, but I kept faith that I would. Faith is everything in the law of attraction, you have to have faith that what you want is going to happen.

I was counting the days, unaware that I was about to learn a very important lesson. The lesson was that things don't always come to you the way you want or when you want. In fact, you can plan things to the smallest detail but something can still happen that changes everything. In these circumstances there is nothing to do but to accept that change is sometimes beyond your control. The journey of life is at times not an easy one, but if you don't have the bad times, would you really be able to appreciate the good times.

I was soon to learn, or, rather, to be reminded, that life can sometimes take a turn in an unexpected way. My friend and I were ready for the tour, bags packed; our excitement high. Then something happened to the band that left the fans unsure if the tour was to go ahead. We waited nervously for news, hoping that all would turn out well.

It's hard to describe what it felt like when the news came out that the tour would be postponed. It was a big disappointment to all those who had tickets, not just to myself. It left me wondering what was going to happen, not only to the tour but also to my project. It was supposed to end on a happy note; I would have met the band.

I walked around the house for a while feeling sorry for myself, not knowing what to do. I had to face a choice; stop the project now and give up or keep the faith and carry on. At the time I was unsure what to do, so I got up and took the dogs for a walk, I find this a good way to clear my head.

By the time I got home I knew what choice I was going to make. The news was a major blow to my project but I still had faith. I had faith in this book and I had faith that my wishes and goals would be achieved. I decided to keep going with the project and have faith that my main wish was going to work out at some point.

The process of the law of attraction had already helped me in dealing with my epilepsy in so many ways. I wasn't prepared to give up yet, after all the tour was only postponed, I still believed that I would meet the band. So what if the project took longer than I thought? The important thing was to have faith that it would happen, after all who said that I was going to meet the band on tour?

With this in mind, I got straight on the phone to my best friend. The hotels had been booked on a cheap non-refundable basis, the train tickets were paid for; we had the time off work. We had a choice, stay at home, mope around or enjoy the moment. We decided to go anyway and have a girl's road trip instead.

We had a wonderful time, involving lots of shopping of course and we made a point of trying new things in every town we visited. We even looked around the venues, not for what we were missing but for what we still had to look forward to. We made the choice not to sit around and think about the tour being postponed but to get on with our lives and enjoy the here and now.

When we got home I realized, apart from taking my medication during the time we were away, I hadn't given the epilepsy a second thought. I couldn't remember the last time that had happened. If I could do that, I could do anything.

Negative Moods

No matter what you do in life or how you try and live, you will come across people who are in a negative state of mind. You can't stop other people being in these moods, though it can be hard for you to stay positive sometimes but you have to be aware that these pessimistic moods can affect you, and, your frame of mind in turn can affect others.

Negative outlooks can affect so much, from how we feel about ourselves, to relationships. They can affect team work and can be destructive to teams. A dispiriting mood can even affect or ruin a complete stranger's day. But we all do it, some perhaps more than others.

Do people realize how their moods can affect others, and do they realize what that effect can be? Do they realize that it can affect how a team works? Someone in a bad mood can put people on edge, would you approach someone for advice or for help if they were giving off those kinds of vibrations? Have you ever walked into a room and could just feel the atmosphere caused by someone in a bad mood and the effect it was having on others?

When I can feel the tension in a room, or hear someone about to lose their temper, I hate it, it makes me on edge. Mainly because I can feel myself almost rising to their level, it's like I'm getting ready for a fight. I have learned to walk away, take some deep breaths and use the event as a reminder to watch my own state of mind, because if someone's mood can affect me, my mood can also affect others. I use it as a reminder to always be nice and pleasant to people no matter what. I like to think that one day my upbeat outlook might just rub off onto someone else.

Some people will avoid working with colleagues who are always in a bad humour; they may even avoid social events or work so that they don't have to be around that person. It's not a nice feeling and the hardest part is not letting the negative rub off onto you when all you want to do is live a positive life.

You need to remember that no matter how badly someone treats you, you should not drop down to their level. You know better and you can just walk away and get on with your own life. You should treat people the way you want to be treated, talk to people the way you want to be spoken to, because respect is earned not given.

Why get into these states? Perhaps things aren't going your way, are you running late for something, perhaps you are tired? Whatever the reason, it's no one's fault and that is what you need to remember. If the trains are running late it's not the ticket guard's fault, so why have a go at him? If you are stuck in a traffic jam is beeping your horn and getting more and more angry going to make things move quicker? You would be better off turning the music up and having a good sing along. It would make a situation you have no control over less stressful. Although personally, I have to make sure the window is closed, as I don't want to scare the other drivers with my singing; but then again, it may give them a laugh. Situations like this you can't do anything about, it's no one's fault, it happens. Try to stop allowing these things to affect you.

When my memory problem occurs and I get caught in mid-sentence, I can see the other person's face getting annoyed, shortly followed by a sigh. This doesn't help me because I find myself getting upset by it, then trying to explain that I have a memory problem because I have epilepsy. Then the person may feel sorry for me and the first conversation is completely forgotten about. I don't want them to feel sorry for me; I just want them to understand.

When this happens I remind myself it's not my fault or theirs, it's something I have to live with and they just don't understand. There is no point in becoming negative or upset. But we can educate people in what it's like to have epilepsy and the possible side effects. The more we get this message out, the more people,

I hope, in time, will understand what it is like.

As always you need to look at ways that your mood may affect others. If you speak in anger you know that the likelihood is that you are going to hurt people's feelings. Then, people may respond in the same way, which will only create a spiral of negative anger.

You can learn to walk away, even if it's only for a few minutes. Get some fresh air or do something else that will help you calm down. Think of your anger as a messenger, look at what is bothering you, what has caused you to feel like this, and look to see what you can do about it, how you can improve things in the future.

When you feel your temper or negativity rising, try some things that might help lift that mood.

- Listen to some uplifting music.
- Think about something that has made you laugh.
- Think about why you have allowed the situation to put you in a bad mood.
- Exercise.
- Have a look around you and appreciate what you have. '
- Accept that we all get into bad moods.
- Try deep breathing exercises.
- If you can, walk away from the situation for a few minutes.
- Accept that people have different views.
- Accept that we cannot control situations, things just happen.

Most importantly, if you do lose your temper, apologize to those involved. Don't construct a chain of negative moods. Show people that you didn't mean what was said or the way in which you said it, don't let them go home worrying, causing sleepless nights, or perhaps passing on your negativity to others.

I confess I'm a worrier. If someone directs something towards me that is not so nice, I will worry about it. Is it something I did, could I have said something differently? In the past I have lost sleep over things like this, only to find out the next day that everything is fine and I worried over nothing.

I don't worry quite so much these days because that negative mood someone is in is down to themselves and for them to sort out. I can be there for them or listen if they need to talk but they will still have to sort out why they are in such a negative state of mind.

When I have had a day of dealing with negative people the first thing I do when I get home is to have a shower. I imagine all the negativity that I picked up during the day just being washed away from me, leaving me with only positive energy. It works; it stops that negative chain of events. That negative chain is what you need to break; instead promote that positive chain; make people feel good about themselves, make people worthwhile. Stop putting people into difficult situations, stop putting people down. Like attracts like, what you do to others will come back to you at some point.

If someone is having a bad day try to be empathetic; why are they having a bad day? Listen to them. Let them get their problems off their chest because once they've talked about the problem it may not seem as bad as they thought. Talking may help to stop them from being negative, stop them from feeling alone. The simple act of giving them your time and allowing them to talk about how they feel could mean more to them than you realize. It's an act of kindness that can go a long way.

Be careful not to take on someone else's negative thoughts. Just listen and be there for them if they need you. You can't change how other people feel, we all have bad days. The important thing is not to let it affect you. If the person is not emotionally connected with you, you can walk away; leave what happened across the day behind. The important thing is not to let your mind go through the events again and again; replaying difficulties and the emotions that they bring about only shows the universe that you want more of the same. When it's a team member that is causing the problem, then that can be a little bit difficult. Perhaps you could try talking to the person, show them what effect they are having on the team or, just simply learn to ignore them.

You also need to remember that it is not only what you say or the vibes you give out that can affect people. It could be your body language, or even through the written word. You can write something, without any intention of upsetting someone, and it can be taken the wrong way. Have you ever sent a text message only to have the recipient take what you've written the wrong way? Similarly, have you ever sent a message written in anger and then later regretted it?

The power of the written word can affect us all more than we perhaps realize and sometimes it can be more hurtful to read something harsh about yourself than being told to your face. When the tour was postponed, fans were all over the social networks having their say. Of course people were upset, we had all lost money through that, but it surprised me that people, for a while, didn't see the reason for the postponement. What scared me though was how quickly I joined in with that negative chain without even thinking about what I was doing. I was feeding off what everyone else was writing. The negative feelings were just fuelling other people's negative reactions.

Once I became aware of what was happening I left the social network sites for a while. Yes, we were all upset about it, but it was getting crazy. When something happens, or when someone's bad mood is affecting you, or maybe you're just having a low day, how do you stop yourself from falling into pessimistic thoughts? You need to quickly turn them into positive thoughts. Otherwise you chance attracting more negative thoughts and negative actions.

You need to remember that your thoughts are powerful, if you allow negative thoughts to dominate, you can become unhappy and you want to be the opposite of this. You need to be aware of your thoughts, because if you allow negative thoughts to carry on, then not only will you be unhappy but all the other steps you have already taken will have been for nothing.

You need to decide that you are no longer going to allow negative thought or negative moods. You decide what your thoughts are and you are the only one who can control what you think. You may not be able to stop negative thoughts popping into your head but you can choose not to listen to them or to push them out of your mind and try to replace them with something more positive.

The next time a negative thought pops into your mind, shrug it off, push it to one side. Change it into a positive thought. But most importantly don't waste your energy or time on worrying about it. Give your energy to positive thoughts and relax.

Learn to stop allowing people and their moods to affect your life. Their mind set is their choice and this is yours. You are in charge of how you feel, today and every day. I'm choosing to be happy.

Situations

All the way throughout life we go through good and bad situations. It could have even been a bad situation that led you to look into the law of attraction as a way to help you through that period of time, just as I discovered the law of attraction when I was first diagnosed with epilepsy. When things are looking bad, don't we all look for help?

When we go through these bad times, can we see a positive outcome? Do we even look? When the road ahead of us looks dark and horrible it's hard to see a way forward, let alone searching for something positive to come out of it.

Too often, and I admit I've been guilty in the past, during a bad situation it is only possible to focus on the negatives. It is understandable to think in terms of 'things aren't going to get any better' or 'why do these things only happen to me'. However, you must learn to step back, take a fresh look at the situation and see what may come from it that could be positive.

Remember the saying 'every cloud has a silver lining'? Perhaps someone has said this to you when you have been in a difficult situation? People often say this to give a person some encouragement when they are facing trying times, in the hope that the person may be able to find something positive in the situation they are in.

As far as I'm concerned it doesn't matter how positive a life we lead, there will always be good times and bad times. There is nothing we can do to change this or to stop it from happening. We can be living the life of our dreams and still go through some bad situations. We may not be able to avoid them but what we can do is change our point of view so when they do happen we don't allow them to be so stressful.

Perhaps see each situation as a lesson and think to yourself, okay, what can I learn from this? Learn your lesson and move on.

Remind yourself that if you didn't have any bad events in your life you wouldn't be able to fully appreciate the good ones.

When I was first diagnosed my world fell apart, I couldn't see a way forward, let alone see anything positive that could come from it. But if I had never had epilepsy what would my life have been like? I would still be plodding along, and for what? Because of my epilepsy I started this project; I'm busy writing this book. Yes, the illness did turn my world upside down but it gave me so much to think about. It opened up my life and showed me there is more to life than working hard. It gave me time to really think about what I truly want out of life and that wasn't where I thought I was heading.

I was so busy thinking about the tour, waiting for the new tour dates, this whole project, that I couldn't believe it was coming up for a year since my last seizure. With some excitement I started the process of applying for my driving licence back. This was a big event for me, a turning point.

I was nervously waiting to see if the DVLA would send it back, so much so that I couldn't do any work on the project. After all, my first wish, made at the very start, was to be seizure free and to be able to drive again and here I was, nervously waiting, wondering if this was when things were going to change. Then, on the 6th August 2011, it arrived. I cried as I opened the letter and held my licence in my hand. Even though I had my licence it took me a while before I braved getting back behind the wheel. I was still a little scared. I had spent so long in fear of having a seizure whilst out in public but the thought of having one whilst I was driving scared me even more. That fear stopped me from driving for a while.

Then I had something else to look forward to. The new tour dates were announced. Time off work was arranged, hotels were re-booked. Then a surprise announcement was made. The band was going to do some special rehearsal dates in the UK; amazing news that lifted the spirits of all the fans. It was going to be an amazing evening that we would never have had if the original tour hadn't been postponed.

I was somewhat nervous as I waited for the screen on the laptop to say I had been lucky in getting two tickets for one of the evening gigs. I just knew the night was going to be amazing and I wasn't wrong. As we made our way home from the event it felt like every time we saw the band we seemed to be getting a little closer each time. It was just a truly amazing night, as I said, one we would never have had if the original tour had gone ahead.

Things were to get even better. A few weeks after this, a work friend was selling her car at a very good price. It was as if it was meant to be because I found the money for it very easily. I just had to buy it; it was time for me to face my fear and get behind that wheel. My first trip home on my own I was so scared but I have never looked back.

Stepping back I could start to see the positive coming out of what had happened, the change in my life since the epilepsy, the rehearsal gigs and there was still more to come. It may be hard at times to stay positive but after a while you should see something and seeing the positive in situations will help you to keep your vibrations high. You need to keep those vibrations high so that you can attract more positive things into your life.

Like attracts like. The more positive you feel, the more positively you view things, the more you will attract positive things into your life.

You need to stop looking at bad news or bad situations and start to look at all the positive things around you. Focus on all the good things that are going on, events, friends and family. To me, it's a shame, because it seems bad news always travels quicker than good news. Yet it's the good news we want to hear and that helps us to remain in our positive mind set.

How Much Work Do We Do?

A question that has been worrying me is – we are doing all this to achieve our dreams but how much work do we do towards our goals? This is another area that confused me concerning the law of attraction. Some books say that working towards our wishes is in fact pushing the wish away.

But is that true? One example I read was of a person who made their vision board about the perfect house they wanted. When it was completed, they put the board away. Years later when they were ready to look for a house, the house that was on the vision board just happened to be available. Just like that, if you want something, it will appear at some point in your life.

Being a person who likes to have control this was quite hard to get my head around. I could understand what was being said, but the thought of not having control over what I wanted was difficult. My own personal view was – how can I sit around and wait for the universe to provide, surely it's not that simple and is there not the possibility that you have to do some ground work to show that you really want this wish?

I mean, all our perfect houses are out there, but they don't just appear. First you need the money to buy the house, or at least to be able to get a mortgage. If you want that dream job, then you need to go out and get the qualifications. If you want to be a bestselling author, then you need to write that book first.

So you can't expect everything to land at your feet without doing some kind of work towards it. Can you expect to get something for nothing?

Surely it's about finding that balance? You can work hard to get the qualifications and leave the universe to help you get the dream job. You can start to save money for your dream house and let the universe do the rest. By doing your part, to me, it's showing the universe that you truly want this and are doing your bit to get to where you want to be. You are making a plan and doing the ground work for your dreams to come true.

This is where the balance comes in. How far do you go to get what you want? You can apply for tons of jobs and keep getting rejection letters and almost give up hope. Then you can look at it in a different manner, you can decide that none of those jobs you applied for are right for you and that the perfect job is around the corner.

I've been there. A while back I wanted to change jobs and applied for several vacancies. And then I applied for more vacancies. The rejection letters just kept coming. I was almost giving up hope that I would find anything; thankfully, I was still in employment so I didn't have to worry about money.

Then I saw something that looked perfect for me but I was in a frame of mind that I wouldn't get it, it was something I had never done before. On the way to the interview I met another person going for the same opening and they had experience in that field where as I had none. Oddly, with this news I found myself relaxing. In my head, that was it, she would get the post. I went to the interview, relaxed, worry free. Two hours later I had a call to say I had the job. That opening led me to gain the qualifications which enabled me to get the job I had always wanted to do.

If that person had not been in the lift that day, I would not have been relaxed about the interview and may never have achieved the position, or the career I have now. Some people do believe that we meet those along our way who can help us to achieve our dreams. I believe this was the case with that interview.

So I'm glad it took a while to find a job and I'm grateful for all those rejection letters because I wouldn't be doing what I love now if I had secured one of the other vacancies. That was my silver lining in that period of my life.

I'm not sure there is a right answer to my question, because there are things you have to do if you want something, but you also have to show trust and have faith that you will get what you want. My own personal view is that you need to do something to work towards your wishes and dreams, finding that balance. I don't think you can just sit back and wait for things to fall into your lap. You should show that you are doing your bit but at the same time you should not be working so hard towards what you want that you are in fact pushing your dreams and wishes away from you.

If I look at my main wish, to meet the band; I have done nothing to achieve this as of yet. I believe it's going to happen and that there is nothing I can do to make it happen. But then, when I say I've done nothing towards this wish, I have in fact bought eight concert tickets and somehow, I think the first time I meet them will be somehow connected with the tour. Time will tell.

You do have to be careful though, because you want to work towards your dreams and not push them away. Even if you are working towards your dreams, you still need to keep faith that the universe is doing its bit to help you gain what you want, and you need to do it in a positive way. Otherwise you risk blocking your wishes. You have to remember that negative thinking and action is the main cause that blocks you from receiving your dreams and that you are the main reason this happens. We are all very quick to assume responsibility for positive events. We're always the cause of success. However, negative things are usually blamed on other people or factors other than ourselves. You need to accept everything in your life and look for the positive in everything.

Without realising it, I believe I blocked this book for a while and this could be one of the reasons it has taken me so long to finish it. When I did the first draft I didn't really believe that the book was good enough. I got friends and family to read it and was always asking what they thought. I got so worried about it that I stopped getting inspiration for it because I stopped believing in myself. I took a break for a few weeks and came back to it because I knew it was the right thing for me, and I hope, for others. We all have it in us to do what we want; we just need to have faith in ourselves and in the universe.

Like attracts like. Negative attracts negative, positive attracts positive. Keep this in mind when you look at things. How you see yourself, your fears, living in the past, being jealous of others, not being patient, the list goes on. If you are negative in this way, then that is what you will attract.

I love hearing stories about people who, against the odds, achieve their hearts desires and I believe it is because they have the right mental attitude. They know what they want; they keep that in mind and go for it. They are positive about their outcome and they succeed in what they set out to achieve. They inspire people because they are not afraid to do what they want and to get what they need. They are living positively and that is where you need to be.

Now is the time to stop blocking yourself. Now is the time to start living. Don't put it off any longer. There is nothing stopping you from living your dream: jobs, money, they are all excuses, they are your blocks. The only thing keeping you from success is yourself. Yes, every single thing you do, no matter how small can take you closer towards your dream. Every decision you make is a step closer to achieving your goals in life.

It takes time, but you will get there. So if you haven't already, get those notebooks and make a list of everything you want out of life. Don't wait until the kids are older, or until you have more money, or till you are seizure free. Start right this minute.

Allow Time

I'm not the most patient person in the world, or should I say I wasn't the most patient person in the world. I lived by the motto 'if I want something, I want it now'. Then I started to live my life using the law of attraction. It was hard at first to be more patient and every now and then I found myself slipping back to my old way of thinking.

Being more patient and allowing my wishes to manifest in their own time is a lot more relaxing than getting stressed because I didn't get that set item at the exact time I wanted it. I'm not sure if I found this difficult initially because I didn't have patience or because living like this meant I didn't have everything under my control.

By being more patient I was also saving money. I didn't realize how much I was spending on things. I would buy items that I wanted at the time and then put them in the cupboard and they would never see the light of day again.

When I wrote my wishes, I didn't want to wait for them. So I gave them a time limit. I have no idea if you can do this with the law of attraction or not. Perhaps you can put a limit on one wish, but was I pushing too hard by putting it on all five? The trouble is, as with a lot of this project, one book would say you could, another would say you shouldn't. I tried setting a deadline and it didn't work.

I now understand that you can't give the universe a time limit, it doesn't have a watch or calendar to work by, it goes with the flow of life. At this point in the project it is six months past the date it was due to be completed. Although I have yet to receive some of my wishes I am seizure free and have my driving licence back. I have had some experiences that I would never have thought I would, so I have faith that the universe knows that I want the experiences and items on my list as soon as possible and I believe that it will provide.

If you really want something you need to keep your mind focused on it and never give up on your dreams. Keep your thoughts positive, relaxed, and focused on your dreams and be patient. You can attract anything you want, but if you want it so badly that the 'not-having' of it causes you anxiety or stress, then that anxiety and stress could be placing you in a negative state, causing you to push your dreams away rather than attract them to you.

So be patient and have faith that your dreams will come about and relax. Don't make long excuses to explain how things are doing at the moment or why your desires have yet to be achieved. By making long excuses you are questioning things, you need to just accept that things will happen when they happen. Everything will come to you at the right moment; you just have to be patient.

It would be nice if all our wishes happened as soon as we asked but as we have already talked about, you cannot giving the universe a deadline and this is where we need to learn patience. I hope that you all get what you want at some point in time; you just need to accept that you can't know when that is going to happen. I like to see it as the fun part, you know it's going to happen, after all that hard work you have done, the ground work is in place, you can now just sit back, relax and wait, knowing that at some point your dreams will come true, it's just a matter of time, and it will make your day when it happens unexpectedly.

Go With The Flow

You need to stop worrying when things are going to happen, you need to be patient and just go with the flow. Going with the flow of life makes things so much easier and our lives so much less stressful. Getting into that frame of mind isn't that easy and can take time. It was hard for me because I like to have control of everything.

We are all so busy these days that going with the flow of life does not seem easy. Our days are taken up with work, with children, walking dogs and endless other matters. The world is already a very stressful place; we don't need to add to the stress, so let's learn to go with the flow.

You must also accept that you can't control everyone or everything. There is no point, whether it's a co-worker, friend, or family member. They are who they are and you are who you are. They are behaving in a way they feel is best for the situation, and would you really want to change them? They are who they are and that is what is wonderful about us humans, we are all different; each one of us has a different interest or way of life. Wouldn't it be boring if we all liked or did the same things?

Not everything in life is what we expect, this is why we need to drop expectations and go with the flow of life. You don't need to stress or strain to make things happen, you can't control what is going to happen, no matter how you may try. If you try and control the outcome you could be missing what the universe is sending your way.

It's okay to plan things, thinking and taking steps for your future is positive; you don't want to become an aimless wanderer. But sometimes you just need to breathe and trust. Let go and see what happens. Trusting and having faith that whatever happens, or whichever way life takes you, it's for the best.

Going with the flow is about accepting that things happen and rolling with the punches. It's about taking what life throws at you and accepting that there is nothing you can do to change the situation.

Try to see the unexpected as a gift. If you miss your train or get stuck in traffic then perhaps there's a reason for that. Perhaps you avoided an accident or ended up meeting someone of interest? Going with the flow is also about making the most of circumstance, even when they are not going your way. You need to seize the moment. Accept that things happen and life doesn't always seem fair.

You are not always going to have what you want. If you had everything what would you have left to work towards? No matter how much structure you create in your life, no matter how many good habits you build, there will always be things that you cannot control. Nobody knows what's going to happen, so why are we so busy trying to plan things? Just look back into your past and think about it. Has past success come from careful planning or did something random come about? A random event that changed your life?

If you let them, these random events can be a huge source of anger, frustration and stress. When you feel yourself getting angry or frustrated take a deep breath, this will help you to calm down and then you can look at the situation again from a calm perspective.

The little things that upset your routine won't matter next week or a year from now, so why get upset about it? You can't change the fact that the trains don't always run on time, or that there is major traffic on the day you are travelling and it makes you late in arriving somewhere. By allowing yourself to get up tight about things, as mentioned before, you could then infect someone else, make them uptight, passing along from one person to another, it could even ruin the day. Your mood can affect other people, just as their mood can affect you.

Sometimes you need to stop worrying about or trying to understand things. Perhaps it's not meant to be understood but accepted. Go where your heart takes you, what feels right for you; stop worrying about things and go with the flow. Going with the flow and not against it can make your life less stressful and difficult.

Believe

One of the most important things when working with the law of attraction is to have faith that your dreams will manifest. But what is more important is to have faith in yourself. You need to know and have faith that you deserve all the good things that are in your life at the moment as well as what is still on its way.

Haven't you ever heard someone say, "I'll believe it when I see it?" Perhaps you've even said it yourself, I know I have. With the law of attraction you believe that what you desire will come to you. But the believing can be the hardest part, yet it's also vital.

When times are hard, things seem to be piling high around you and you can't see the path ahead of you, you still need to believe in your dreams. Because all the steps, focusing your thoughts and emotions and taking action to manifest your dreams, all this is pointless if you don't believe in yourself or don't believe your dreams will materialize.

Having this kind of faith helps you to keep focused, even through the tough times. I know it's not always easy and when I first started reading about the law of attraction I did say to myself, "Crazy people." It's not easy to keep that belief going when you feel like the world is against you. With the depression I had from my last seizure I couldn't see a way forward. I even almost gave up, but something inside me kept me going. Have faith that what you focus on will grow, so let the positive grow in your life and watch your dreams become reality.

When the tour was postponed the project was up in the air. Even now, after the delay in completing the book, I still have firm faith that I will meet the band. You need to believe in yourself, believe that you are worth it and will gain your dreams. This belief will give you strength to carry on when times are hard.

If you don't believe something is going to change in your life, nothing will. So stop those negative thoughts and accept things can change, change is possible. Make plans, talk about them and write them in your journal.

Let yourself believe – it is possible, you can do it, and it is happening.

Using things like the vision boards is a great way to help you see what it is you need, use your imagination. Plus, feel what it is you want. Believing that what you desire will come to you is perhaps the hardest thing. You need to fully believe that your dream is on its way and it is going to happen. I have been told that this is where most people lose their desire, because they don't truly believe that what they want will be achieved.

With the first draft of this book I asked friends and family to read bits as I was going along. Thinking back on it, was I in fact decreasing the energy of the wishes? Not only that, I now realize I didn't have enough faith in myself. I needed other people's opinions to verify the worth of my work. You could say I had lost faith in myself.

You need faith in yourself, and in the universe, in order for your wishes to be drawn to you. Don't question how that's going to happen, believe that it will. One day you may be that best-selling author or you may meet the people you so desire. It's all out there; you just need to have faith.

Whether or not you believe in the universe to provide doesn't matter. At the end of the day, if you don't believe in yourself, who's going to believe in you?

Never Ever Say Never

Never ever, ever, say never. The more I work with the law of attraction, the more it saddens me when I hear people say, "It's never going to happen to me." Of course, that was me a few years ago but I can now safely say it can happen. As soon as you say never, you've lost faith in yourself and in your dreams. Nothing is impossible and people can do things that they thought they never would be able to. When you think like this, are you missing the opportunities that could be right in front of you? Opportunities that could help you to fulfil your dreams.

You only have one life...Follow your dreams, have faith in your dreams, and never say never.

When I first started this project, to be honest, I wasn't truly sold on the law of attraction. I was in a place where I hadn't yet accepted that I had epilepsy. I hadn't really accepted the changes that were happening to me, changes that I had no control over.

There are no obstacles so big that with the right support you cannot overcome them. Once you realize just how big an impact your words can have on your happiness you will never want to say never again. Life is to be enjoyed, focus on the positive not the negative. The word 'never' is such a negative word. Anything can happen if you truly want it.

Having re-read this book there have been many amazing events, as well as a few pitfalls, along the way and that is the joy of life. Apart from a couple of times, I never gave up hope, I held onto that hope that my dreams would come true.

The big question is – did I get my dream? Did I get to meet the band? We now had our new tour dates, hotels were booked and we were packed, ready to go. This time around we were only going to seven of the concerts. We had to sell some of our tickets because I couldn't get all the time off work that I needed for the new dates. That was not a problem; I was more than happy with the seven I could make. Those seven dates turned out to be truly memorable events in my life, ones I shall make sure I never forget.

When the tour was first postponed we had a choice and we decided to go on a girl's road trip. I don't know why, but we went to the venues in each town we visited and had a little look around. Each venue had its posters up saying, 'concert postponed'. Oddly it didn't get us down; perhaps because we knew that the band would be touring again, and soon. We were to find out that these little tours of the venues were going to work for our benefit. Why? Because without realizing it then we were able to use information we had gathered when the new tour opened. You could say that for that one, short time, we became stalkers.

At the first concert we saw a few people hanging around the stage door. We had never done this before, but there's a first time for everything. At the end of the concert we waited with the rest of the fans, and then, the band came out. We were closer to them than we had ever been before and the excitement was amazing. At that moment I felt it was only a matter of time.

At the second concert we did the same. Although we didn't meet the band, we did meet some lovely people.

Then it happened! At the third concert we met two of the band members, had photos taken with them and got their autographs. Oh, the feeling was amazing!

The excitement carried us into the fourth concert, where we met two more of the band members and at the fifth concert we met the final member. The excitement of all this happening was incredible and I don't think I slept that night, and perhaps I should say sorry to my husband and parents for phoning them at some crazy hour to tell them we had done it; we had met the entire band.

The sixth date we don't talk about and by the seventh date we were happy with what we had achieved and enjoyed our last concert. We had done it! We had met the band! A lifelong dream completed and the ultimate, amazing wish for this project achieved. It was wonderful to finally say I had met the band that I have followed since I was a child.

The meetings were brief, that aside, we did meet them. We spent a lot of time before and after the concerts waiting outside stage doors. Even now I can't quite believe we did that and I don't think at the time I could quite believe we were doing it having never done anything like that before.

I can say I've done it now. Although I don't think I'll be repeating the experience. Waiting around outside venues was good fun, although I wish they had toured in the spring months then I wouldn't have been so cold. On the plus side I met the band and came away without a cold.

It's true it didn't happen the way I expected or wanted. It was an experience, and one I will never forget. If it had happen the way I visualised I would not have met some wonderful people along the way, people who have remained friends to this day. And I like to see this experience as a warm up to meeting them again, although perhaps in the warmth this time. So far this project has been an amazing journey and I have completed one of my life wishes.

My story is not over yet, there are still wishes to come. One is to win a competition; another is to get this book published. Concerning the competition, I've entered a few, even entered a few for getting this book published. As of yet, I haven't won anything, I will, like everything it's a matter of time.

This isn't a negative thought and I think it's healthy to question things, but surely the more competitions you enter, the more you increase your chance of winning something? The question is do you win something for the sake of winning, or do you win something because it helps you to gain your dream? I haven't gone out of the way to enter lots of competitions; just the ones that would help me manifest my dream.

We know that life isn't always perfect but it's what you make of it. Sometimes you have to stop worrying, wondering and doubting. Have faith that things will work out, maybe not how you planned, but how it's meant to be.

So make it count, make it memorable and never let anyone steal your happiness. Most importantly, never say never.

Final Thoughts

This journey I have been on has been amazing. My life before the epilepsy was career driven, more to the point, it was mostly about how much money I could earn doing extra shifts. The more money I could get, the more material stuff I could buy. I lived in a world where second hand was not an option when I could get it shiny and new.

Then I developed epilepsy, and this may sound crazy to some, but I give thanks for that. Not being given the choice and having to slow down has shown me there is so much more to life than chasing money. I think about it now and wonder how much I may have missed out on because I was so busy looking to see how I could make more to spending on things that really didn't make me happy.

This journey has shown me a whole new life and I will never look back. I have learned so very much along the way. Below is a list of some of what I view now as being of primary importance:

- Figure out what it is I really want out of life.
- Say something nice.
- Choose love.
- Plan my next steps carefully but also be able to go with the flow of life.
- Laugh more.
- Give thanks.
- Use my vision board to see what I now want out of life.
- Think positively.
- Avoid the blame game.
- Be the victor, not the victim.
- Use affirmations.
- Do good deeds.
- Forgive myself and others.

- Get excited.
- Live in the now.
- Not take things for granted.
- See the unexpected as a gift.
- Stop letting my fear control my life and hold me back.

One of the biggest realizations I've made is that you can't live your life the way others think you should, according to what they think is right. It's not going to make you happy because that person they want you to be isn't the person you are. Only really being yourself will make you happy. Being happy will make you feel good and make those who truly love you happy also. Being happy is such a positive thing and of major importance in achieving your goals.

My epilepsy made me take a good, hard, look at my life. It showed me I wasn't that happy. The law of attraction has helped me to deal with the illness. It has helped me to deal with what was happening to me and in coming to terms with this disorder. It has helped me to see that no matter how I felt, there was a future out there for me and it gave me the strength to get up and go out and get it.

So this is my journey, my journey of living and dealing with epilepsy. If you haven't started already, now is the time for you to start yours. You are never too young or old to set new goals, or to dream a new dream.

Out of all this I hope to help raise awareness of epilepsy to help people to understand what it's like. To possibly help those who have this disorder and to help family and friends who want to support a loved one who has epilepsy.

Don't give up, once you are prepared to embrace change and believe from the heart, the world is your oyster. For me this is just the start of my new journey, let it be the start of your new journey, a journey to a wonderful and happy life, full of joy and love with all your dreams coming true.

Soul Rocks is a fresh list that takes the search for soul and spirit mainstream. Chick-lit, young adult, cult, fashionable fiction & non-fiction with a fierce twist